···MOMMYBOPS···SACK OF ANGRY RABBITS···TA-TAS···TITS···THE GIRLS···THE TODDLERS···
ND ROY···GIN AND TONIC···TH   AND PA
D FRUTTI···HOSS AND LITTLE   L··
2···BABALOOS···BABY FEED   OK
S···BILLIBONGS···BLINKERS··   OB
··CANTALOUPES···CHA-CHAS   S···
UMPLINGS···DURANTES···EA   DOODLES···FR   ET
··GOODYEARS···GOOMBAS···   IGHTS···HIGH BEAMS···HO
··JAHOOBIES···JOHN AND P   NGAS···KNOCKERS···LEWI
NNIE···MIKE AND IKE···MILK B   MILKMAKERS···MILKSHA
·NUM-NUMS···PAIR···PALOOKAS···PIA ZADORAS···PILLOWS···PUPPIES···PUSHMATAHAS···RA
SPEED BUMPS···SPLAZOINGAS···SQUACHIES···TATAS···TEETEES···THELMA AND LOUISE···TI
OLVOS···WAHWAHS···WHIMWHAMS···WILSONS···WINDSHIELD WIPERS···WINNEBAGOS···W
HESTICLES···JUBBLIES···JUG-A-LUGS···KNOCKERS···MOMMYBOPS···SACK OF ANGRY RABBIT
GISTRATION···LUCY AND ETHEL···SIEGFRIED AND ROY···GIN AND TONIC···THELMA AND LO
AND BITTY···HANDEL AND MOZART···TUTTI AND FRUTTI···HOSS AND LITTLE JOE···BEN AN
··ABBOTT AND COSTELLO···AIRBAGS···B1 AND B2···BABALOOS···BABY FEEDERS···BADOIN
JERRY···BERT AND ERNIE···BERTHAS···BIJONGAS···BILLIBONGS···BLINKERS···BOB AND RAY
DERS···BRAD PITTS···BRISTOLS···BUMPERS···CANS···CANTALOUPES···CHA-CHAS···CHESTIC
TH··DEVIL'S DUMPLINGS···DINGLEBOBBERS···DUGS···DUMPLINGS···DURANTES···EARTHA K
·GOBSTOPPERS···GOD'S MILK BOTTLES···GODZILLAS···GOODYEARS···GOOMBAS···GRILLW
·HOOTERS···HUBCAPS···HUMMERS···ISAAC NEWTONS···JAHOOBIES···JOHN AND PAUL···JU
·MAMMARIES···MAU MAUS···MELONS···MICKEY AND MINNIE···MIKE AND IKE···MILK BOMBS··
URPHYS···NAY-NAYS···NEENERS···NINNIES···NORKS···NUM-NUMS···PAIR···PALOOKAS···PIA
SHLOBES···SHMOZOBS···SNOW TIRES···SOOMBAS···SPEED BUMPS···SPLAZOINGAS···SQUA
E AND TWEEDLEDUM···TWEETERS···TWEKKERS···VOLVOS···WAHWAHS···WHIMWHAMS···W
··BOOBIES···BRESTICLES···CHESTICLES···JUBBLIES···JUG-A-LUGS···KNOCKERS···MOMMYB
UBERANCES···LICENSE AND REGISTRATION···LUCY AND ETHEL···SIEGFRIED AND ROY···GI
WEETY AND SYLVESTER···ITTY AND BITTY HANDEL AND MOZART···TUTTI AND FRUTTI···H
AND DALE··THE SUPERHEROES···ABBOTT AND COSTELLO···AIRBAGS···B1 AND B2···BABAL
BAS···BEE-STINGS···BEN AND JERRY···BERT AND ERNIE···BERTHAS···BI   LIBON
BOSOMS···BOTTLES···BOULDERS···BRAD PITTS···BRISTOLS···BUMPERS···CANS···CANTALO
VITOS···DAVID AND GOLIATH···DEVIL'S DUMPLINGS···DINGLEBOBBERS···DUGS···DUMPLIN

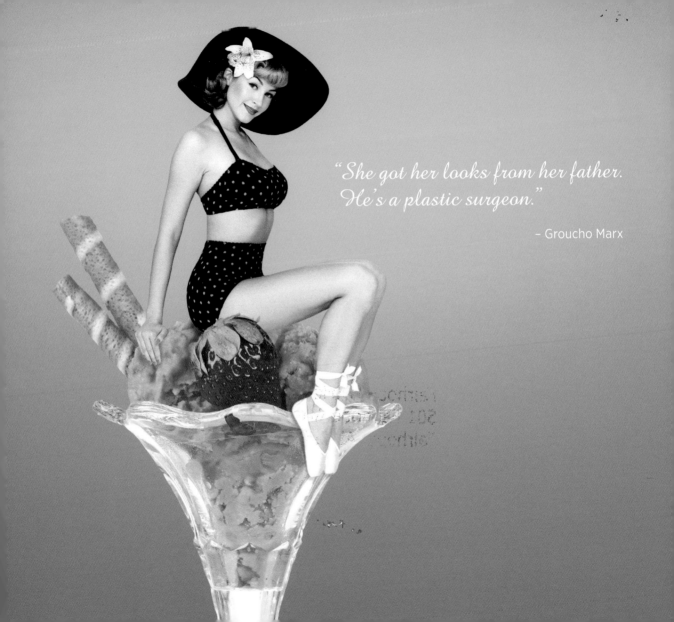

"She got her looks from her father.
He's a plastic surgeon."

– Groucho Marx

The Scoop on Breasts

A PLASTIC SURGEON BUSTS THE MYTHS

Dr. Ted Eisenberg

Joyce K. Eisenberg

incompra press

Book Design by Sara Hodgson and Anoki Casey
www.incompra.com

For a complete list of photo and illustration credits,
turn to page 187.

ISBN-13: 978-0-9857249-0-0

Printed by ANRO Inc. in the United States of America

The information contained in this book represents the opinions
of Dr. Ted Eisenberg, based on his training, experience and
observations, and is for general interest only; other physicians
may have different opinions. No information found here should
be construed as personal medical advice or instruction and
should not be used as a substitute for consultation with
practicing medical professionals.

DEDICATION

To my wife, my staff and my patients,
who have taught me that my job is just to listen.

Thank you for your trust in me and
for giving me the opportunity
to make a difference in your lives.

– T. E.

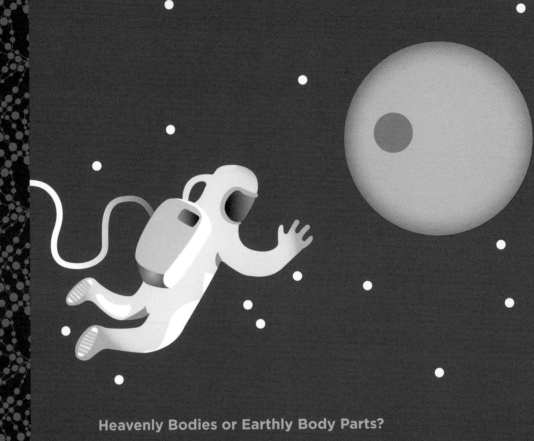

Heavenly Bodies or Earthly Body Parts?

Stedman's Medical Dictionary defines breast as "one of two **large hemispheric projections** situated in the subcutaneous tela over the pectoralis major muscle on either side of the chest." Maybe that's why so many earthlings consider breasts to be heavenly bodies.

TABLE OF CONTENTS

For a complete list of questions by chapter,
turn to page 188.

Acknowledgments

I'm a lucky guy. I'm surrounded by angels.

I am blessed by the love of my wife, Joyce. She has nurtured me through college, medical school, surgical residencies, and years of practice. She has listened to all my stories, laughed at all my jokes, and shared my excitement about my work. She is a terrific partner, whether we are parenting, ballroom dancing, or writing together. I am grateful to her for bringing this book from concept to reality.

I am so fortunate to work every day with Eileen Ricciutti, Nan McCarthy, Sharon Sisle, Gerry Gorgol and Pat Smith. They treat each woman who walks through our door as if she were their daughter or their sister. They receive love notes from patients daily, and they deserve every compliment they get. Without my dedicated and enthusiastic staff, I couldn't do what I do, which includes writing this book. They kept lists of the questions that patients asked, shared their experiences in the office, reviewed the manuscript, and contributed to it considerably.

My deep appreciation goes to my children, both of whom are skilled writers. My son, Ben, contributed fun facts to this book and kept me on my toes by questioning data, requesting sources, and recommending less use of the word "I." He has been a great source of marketing ideas as well as my social media guru. Thanks to him, you can follow our tweets at #ScoopOnBreasts. Like my patients, my daughter, Samantha, grew up with a barrage of media messages about beauty, dieting and body image. She made sure that I was sensitive to – and politically correct about – these issues; her insightful comments and careful reading helped me clarify passages that were confusing.

I am indebted to Sara Hodgson and Anoki Casey, the visual architects of this book who, like Cinderella's fairy godmother, waved a magic wand over the manuscript to dress it up and bring it to life. They are responsible for the book design and the illustrations. I am honored to be their client and their friend.

When I told my friends that I was writing a book about cosmetic breast surgery, they couldn't resist making suggestions for chapter titles and illustrations. Thanks to all of them, but especially to Nathan Wright, R.C. Atlee, Janis Traven and Mark Linsey, whose clever suggestions made the final cut and helped enhance the manuscript.

I thank my parents, Marty and Mitzi, for giving me the opportunity and supporting my decision to go to medical school.

Early on, my brother Ron, a family physician, shared two bits of advice with me: "Work hard. The cream rises to the top" and "All that matters in life is that you are happy where you go to in the morning and where you come home to at night." His wise counsel has stayed with me through the years.

I have long been in awe of my brother Barry's artistic talent. His imagination and creativity have inspired me to think outside the box. He is an artist who chose to become a family doctor; I like to think that in my practice of cosmetic surgery I am an artist as well.

Nazareth Hospital has given me another home away from home. I am thankful to the dedicated staff in the Operating Room, PACU and SPU, and to the members of the Anesthesia Department. They provide compassionate care to my patients and skilled assistance to me so that I can do my job efficiently and seamlessly. It's teamwork at its best.

I am indebted to Dr. Murray Seitchik, my plastic surgery mentor, for giving me the opportunity to learn by his side. He taught me sound fundamentals and plastic surgery principles that I could rely on when I faced surgical challenges during my career – when I reconstructed a nose lost to cancer or created a new approach to simultaneous breast augmentation and lift.

I would not be the surgeon I am today without the guidance of the following doctors:

Michael Abraham, Charles Benjamin, Al Bonier, Dominic Bontempo, Allan Fields, Len Finkelstein, Ron Ganelli, Jim Hunter, Jay Joseph, Stan Kaye, Ernest Manders, Anthony Minissale, Julius Newman, Barrett Noone, Nicholas Pedano, Jane Petro, Thomas Powell, Larry Schneider, Marshall Shapiro, Mel Shiffman, David Silverman, Ed Silverman, Richard Smialek, Scott Spear, Wynne Steinsnyder and Daniel Wisely.

Finally, my heartfelt thanks goes to all the women who have chosen me to be their doctor and whose questions inspired the subject matter of this book.

We are BBF: Bosom Buddies Forever.

  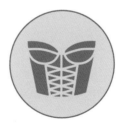  

Introduction

At a party or at the gym, it is invariably the men who ask me what I do for a living. When I reply "cosmetic breast surgery," the questions follow: Do you get a lot of exotic dancers? Does your wife mind that you look at other women's breasts all day? Can I be your assistant? Does your wife have implants?

In brief: No. No. No. None of your business.

Women are not as public with their questions. But on the phone with one of my staff members or in the privacy of a consultation, they ask what they want to know: Am I too old for breast augmentation? Will implants boil in a hot tub? Do they need to be replaced every 10 years? Does your wife have implants?

In brief: No. No. No. None of your business.

Through the years, my staff and I kept a list of the questions most commonly asked and the ones that tickled us: questions about bulletproof vests, bags of birdseed, and kickboxing. After thousands of consultations and tens of thousands of questions, I thought, "I could write a book."

I didn't have to go far to find a co-author. My wife, Joyce, has a successful career as an author and editor, and through the years she has lent her writing talents to my website content, radio and TV ads, and press releases. I knew that her research, writing, editing and organizational skills would keep this project on track, and I also knew that we would have fun writing a book together. I was right on both counts.

The Scoop on Breasts is an attempt to answer these questions in an educational and entertaining way and to bust some of the myths about breast implants and the women who get them. I have tried to present accurate medical information based on the latest data. I have also aimed to be "fair and impartial," as they say, but I'm not really impartial: After doing 5,000 breast augmentations, I have a point of view about the best approach and opinions about what can and cannot be accomplished. If you were to ask another plastic surgeon these same questions, you might get different answers.

. . . .

When I was a child, I never dreamed I would grow up to be a cosmetic breast surgeon. Sure, like many of my middle school buddies, I was interested in breasts. Seeing them – and getting to "second base" – did occupy some of my time, but I was no more interested in breasts than Steve, who went to work for NASA, or David, who became a university dean. I liked math, and then I discovered mechanical drawing. I loved the detail, the exactness, the way I could draw something in two dimensions that could be realized in three. I thought I might become an architect.

By 11th grade, with college looming, the pressure was on to decide what I wanted to be when I grew up. Both of my brothers were family practitioners, and I thought it would be fun to become a doctor and have a *family* family practice with them. I went to Penn State and majored in pre-med.

During my internship following medical school, I discovered that I was good with my hands and that my best aptitude was in surgery. I am a tactile learner. When I did physical examinations during my obstetrical rotation, I was as good as an ultrasound machine at determining how many weeks pregnant a woman was. Before I could consider a career in obstetrics and gynecology, I was smitten with plastic surgery: I attended a lecture on rhinoplasty (nose jobs), and I was fascinated by the before-and-after photos and the significant and immediate changes that surgery made.

I became a plastic and reconstructive surgeon, and for 14 years I did everything from head to toe. I was a pioneer with tissue expanders: I used them to reconstruct a nose lost to cancer and a scalp shredded by shrapnel. I rebuilt an eye socket damaged by radiation so that a young woman could have an artificial eye on her wedding day. I was an architect of the body.

Fast-forward to 1999. I asked myself a hypothetical question along the lines of: If I could eat only one kind of food for the rest of my life, what would it be? (I'd pick pizza.) The question was this: If I could perform only one surgery all day, every day, what would it be? My answer was breast augmentation. I was very good at it, and I loved seeing the immediate results. I liked the idea of becoming an expert in one aspect of plastic surgery – cosmetic breast surgery. I took the plunge, which meant turning away women who wanted liposuction or nose jobs. It was the right choice for me.

Since then, I have focused my practice entirely on cosmetic breast surgery. I am not bored, even for a minute. People ask me that, too. I'm the kind of guy who likes to focus on – and stick with – one thing at a time:

- My wife: I have been married to Joyce for 38 years. We met when she was 17 and I was 18.

- My sneakers: I have bought the same style (or as close as I can get when they update the line) for the last 15 years.

- My food: I eat one thing at a time on my dinner plate – not a little bite of this and a little bite of that.

- My hobby: Tournament knife throwing involves hurling the same knife at the same target over and over again. In three years, I have progressed from novice to expert. I've also earned a nickname: **The Boobinator.**

I want to be the best: the best husband, the best surgeon, the best boss, the best knife thrower. This quest started early. I was the third of three sons. My parents expected that I would do as well and accomplish as much as my two older brothers did, but I wanted to do better and do more.

I wanted to be the No. 1 son. That's why I am proud to hold a Guinness World Record for the most breast augmentation surgeries performed in a lifetime. My brothers don't have that honor!

When I look back, it seems as if the pieces of the puzzle have fallen into place. Perhaps it's destiny. My paternal grandfather, Tobias, for whom I am named, was a tailor who immigrated to America from Poland. Sometimes when I am sewing an incision closed, I think of him. I believe he would have been proud of "Teddy the Titty Tailor," a nickname bestowed upon me by a British nurse.

After doing so many breast surgery consultations, I have gained the following insights:

- There is no stereotypical cosmetic breast surgery patient. My patients range in age from 18 to 63 and come from all walks of life. Only a tiny percentage of them are exotic dancers.

- Women want to look natural and proportional. They want their clothes to fit better. They want to recapture what they lost after pregnancy or weight change.

- Breasts are sisters, not twins. In consultation, when women look at dozens of before-and-after photos, they are surprised and relieved to see that they are not the only one with different-sized breasts.

- Women know what they want. During medical training, we are taught that we should know the answers, that we are the authority. But I have discovered that women know best. My job is to listen carefully and to determine if there is a match between their goals and what I can accomplish. I believe I am an expert at figuring that out.

- I don't pass women on the street and think they need my services. I don't believe there is an ideal breast size and then impose it on my patients. And I know that cosmetic breast surgery is not for everyone. Two women could look alike in terms of breast size and shape, and while one might be perfectly happy, the other might want to make a change.

For those women who choose cosmetic breast surgery, the change can be profound. I am moved, often to tears, when a woman expresses her feelings about the difference surgery has made for her – in person or in a thank-you note like this one:

Dear Dr. Eisenberg and Staff,

Today was my final checkout after my breast augmentation, and I just have to tell you again how I feel. The surgery has given me a confidence I never had before. Basically I am the same person – just a new and improved version. I actually feel good in my skin.

I used to hate lingerie and bathing suit shopping. Now I love it. In fact, all my old bathing suits looked brand new this summer. I have gotten many "You look great" comments.

I would say I wish I had done this years ago, but my daughter was a teenager then and I wasn't sure about the message it might send to her. I also thought being flat-chested was my badge of honor or courage. I told myself, "This is who I am. I'm better than that."

Being flat-chested didn't stop me from developing into a confident, intelligent, caring and giving person. That has not changed, but now I just feel so much better. A burden that I had been thinking about has been lifted. It is a newfound freedom.

My marriage has never been better, and it keeps getting better. It is not just the intimacy, which is beyond what we ever thought it could be, but also our communication and how we treat each other.

I tell everyone who is considering cosmetic breast surgery to go for it, and I will always tell them to go to you.

With my deepest appreciation . . .

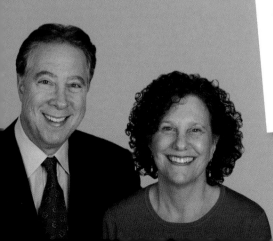

The Authors: Ted and Joyce Eisenberg

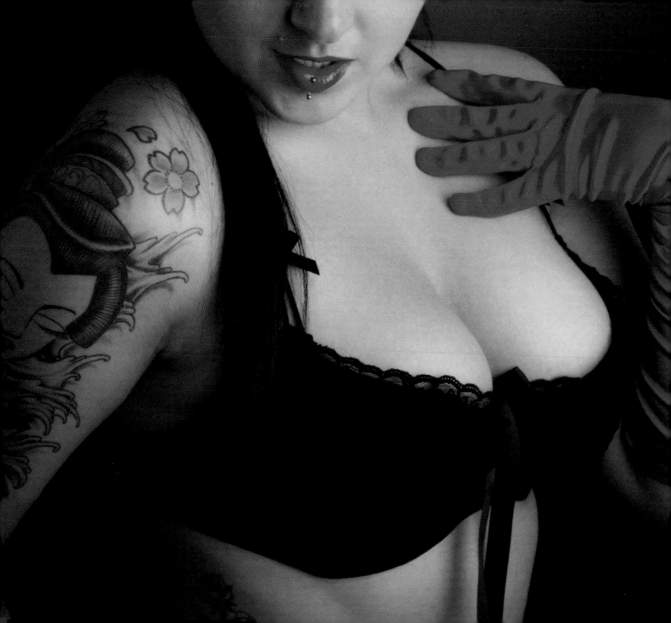

Chapter 1

A Tale of Two Titties

*"It was the breast of times, it was the worst of times,
it was the age of wisdom, it was the age of foolishness ..."*

In keeping with the spirit of Charles Dickens,
we are bringing you both wisdom
and foolishness about breasts.
There is no better place to begin our tale
than with booby basics –
the who, what, where, when and why of developing.

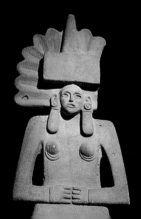

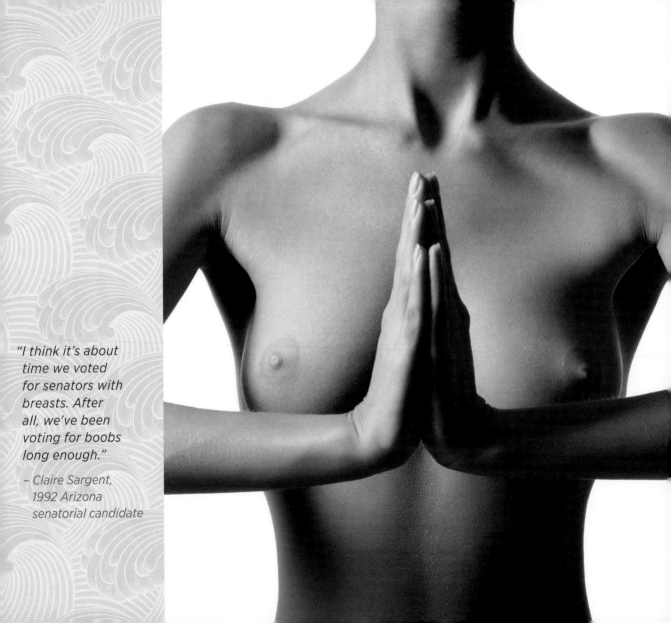

"I think it's about
time we voted
for senators with
breasts. After
all, we've been
voting for boobs
long enough."

— Claire Sargent,
 1992 Arizona
 senatorial candidate

What's in a breast?

Breasts are not made just of sugar and spice and everything nice. The breast of an adult female is a milk-producing gland. Here's what you'll find beneath the surface:

- Glandular tissue, which contains lobules (milk-producing glands) and ducts that deliver the milk from the glands to openings in the nipple.

- Fatty tissue, which surrounds the lobules and ducts and extends throughout the breast. This fatty tissue gives the breast its size, shape and softness.

- Connective tissue, which supports the breast and helps maintain its shape.

- The nipple and the surrounding pigmented skin, known as the nipple-areola complex (NAC). It is made of erectile tissue containing sensory nerves, which are sensitive to touch and to cold.

- A network of capillaries (thin blood vessels), which allows oxygen and nutrients to travel to the breast tissue.

Immediately beneath the breast but not part of it are the pectoralis major and pectoralis minor muscles.

When do breasts start growing?

They get an early start – in utero. About six weeks after conception, a ridge of breast tissue begins to develop in a line that runs from the axilla (armpit) to the groin. It's called the milk ridge. Over the next several months, cells begin to organize themselves into lobules, and the nipple-areola complex begins to form. Boys and girls have exactly the same breast structure until puberty.

Why do girls seem to mature so much earlier than boys?

Because they actually do. In general, girls get a head start on puberty by about one or two years. Since the first physical sign of puberty in girls is breast development, they mature more publicly than boys, whose first physical sign is testicular enlargement.

Breast development is triggered by the body's production of estradiol, one of three naturally occurring estrogens in women. Growth begins with a breast bud, a little button containing fat, tissue and milk glands, which makes the nipple stick out from the chest. Soon, the areola slightly increases in size. The process can start first on one side or on both sides at the same time. It takes about three to five years for the glandular tissue to fully develop and for breasts to reach their full adult size. Girls usually first menstruate 2 to 2½ years after the breast buds appear.

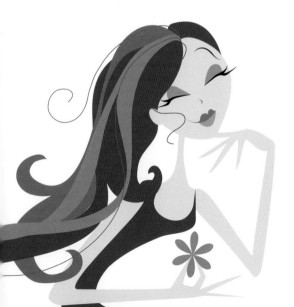

⊙⊙ Titbit: While menarche is the term for the first menstrual cycle, thelarche is the term for breast development. It comes from the Greek words for "nipple" and "beginning."

⊙⊙ Titbit: A bloomer is a plant that produces flowers at a specific time. "Early bloomer" is a term for a girl who develops more quickly than her peers. Perhaps the term alludes to the fact that breast buds are the first sign of development.

▶ Are girls developing earlier these days?

Yes. Many young girls are not just acting and dressing like grown-ups; they really are growing up earlier – physically. According to the authors of a 2010 article in the journal *Pediatrics*, the age of onset of puberty has fallen in the past two decades. They reported that at age 7, approximately 10 percent of white girls, 23 percent of black girls, and 15 percent of Hispanic girls had breast development.

The childhood obesity epidemic gets much of the blame: Body fat is a key player in the production of estrogens, and estrogens trigger puberty. In Scandinavia in the 1840s, the average age at first menstruation was 16 to 17. Because of poor nutrition and infectious diseases, girls were very thin; endocrinologists think this lack of fat sent a message to the body that it was not ready to carry a pregnancy. As diet and living conditions improved, the age at first menstruation moved up two to three months each decade. In the United States in 2010, the average age for a girl to get her first period was 12.

◉ ◉
Titbit
The human female is the only mammal whose breasts develop
and stay enlarged throughout her life. Other mammals,
such as chimpanzees, dogs and cats, have swollen breasts
only during pregnancy and lactation.

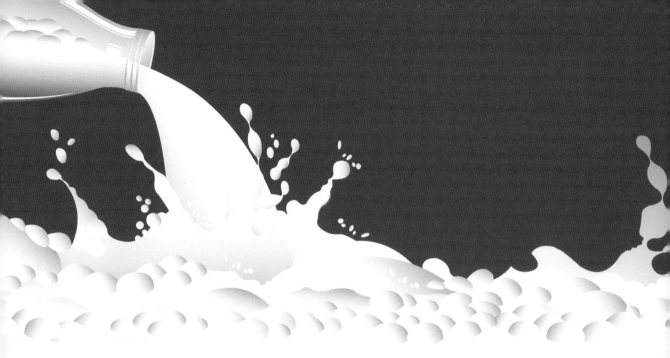

▶ Will drinking milk make my boobs grow?

Milk treated with protein hormones has been suspected of contributing to early puberty, but no link has been proven. In a 1993 report, which was reaffirmed in 2009, the U.S. Food and Drug Administration (FDA) determined that food products from cows treated with rbGH (recombinant bovine growth hormone) are safe for consumption by humans. The report stated that "the proteins typically are broken down in the digestive process and are not absorbed into the body."

Other reasons for what's called "precocious puberty" may be premature birth, genetics, and exposure to plastics and insecticides, which can break down into chemicals that are similar to estrogens.

Do I need to wear a bra?

No, but I am answering as your doctor, not your mother.
A bra will keep your breasts from sagging, but only while you are
wearing it. There's little evidence that wearing a bra delays or prevents breast
droopiness or the formation of stretch marks. Bras do serve a few purposes, though.

*Shape and lift: Manhattan dressmaker Ida Rosenthal didn't like the boyish flapper style
that was popular in the 1920s, for which women wore side-lacing bras to flatten their
breasts. To make her feminine styles fit right, she sewed in a band with two cups that
accentuated and supported the breasts. When clients began to request separate bras,
Rosenthal, along with her husband, William, and her business partner, Enid Bisset,
decided to manufacture their bras under the brand name of Maiden Form; in 1928,
they sold 500,000 bras.*

*Comfort: Women with large breasts say the straps and elastic of
a well-made bra can take some of the weight off their shoulders
and back. Bras can also prevent uncomfortable bouncing when
you exercise or play a sport.*

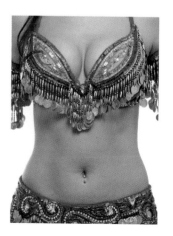

*Convenience: Bras make a great place to stash your stuff when you
go clubbing. Women report that they have put cash, credit cards, car
keys, driver's licenses, lip gloss, gum, condoms and phones in their
bras. Entertainers tuck tips into their bra straps. Some women have
memories of their grandmothers stashing Kleenex in their bras, not
to increase their bust size but to be ready for any emergency.*

These coconut shell flopper stoppers are fun to look at but uncomfortable to wear.

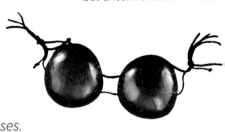

The First Chicken Cutlet

In Victorian England in the mid-1800s, girls were considered adults at the age of 15. If they had not developed enough to fit into the women's clothing they were supposed to wear, they were given bosom pads to fill out the bodices of their dresses.

The First Sports Bra

The Minoan civilization thrived on the island of Crete from 2700-1400 B.C. The women are generally depicted wearing robes open to their waists, leaving their breasts exposed, but in illustrations that portray them engaged in the ritual sport of bull-leaping, they are wearing bra-like garments.

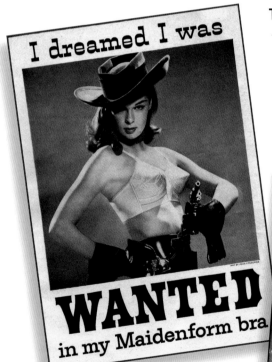

I dreamed I was

WANTED

in my Maidenform bra

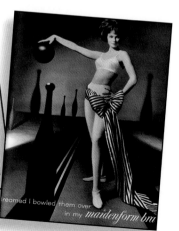

I dreamed I bowled them over in my *maidenform bra*

Maidenform got sporty with its risqué "I Dreamed" campaign, launched in 1949. Models, wearing only a bra from the waist up, dreamed they were toreadors and tightrope walkers, bowlers and ballerinas.

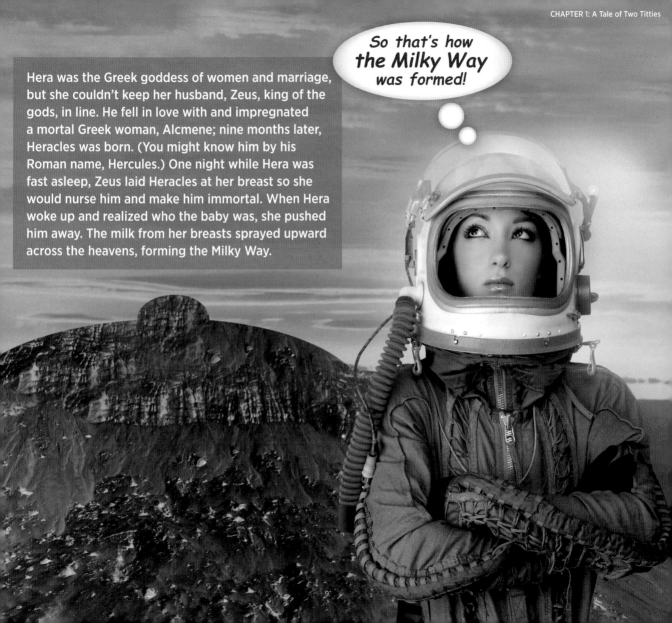

So that's how **the Milky Way** was formed!

Hera was the Greek goddess of women and marriage, but she couldn't keep her husband, Zeus, king of the gods, in line. He fell in love with and impregnated a mortal Greek woman, Alcmene; nine months later, Heracles was born. (You might know him by his Roman name, Hercules.) One night while Hera was fast asleep, Zeus laid Heracles at her breast so she would nurse him and make him immortal. When Hera woke up and realized who the baby was, she pushed him away. The milk from her breasts sprayed upward across the heavens, forming the Milky Way.

Why do I have stretch marks?

Skin and rubber bands have similar properties: If you stretch a rubber band a little bit and let it go, it will snap back to its original shape. If you pull it too far or stretch it out over and over again, it will break. Overstretched skin acts much the same way. When the body grows faster than the skin can stretch – during puberty, pregnancy, or from a quick weight gain – the elastic fibers in the dermis tear and show up as stretch marks, or striae.

Most women have stretch marks, commonly on their hips, thighs and breasts. The marks start out as red or purple lines and usually fade to skin color over time.

If I use a lot of lotion, will it prevent stretch marks?

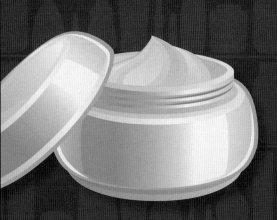

There is no definitive medical proof that creams and lotions prevent or eliminate stretch marks; they don't penetrate to the dermis, the layer of skin between the epidermis and the subcutaneous tissue where stretch marks occur. Skin does crave moisture, and moisturizing lotions can help the appearance and itchiness of stretch marks, so consider using lotion like eating chicken soup when you have a cold: It can't hurt.

But Skipper Didn't Get Stretch Marks …

Hot Stuff Skipper had dimples and Malibu Skipper had waist-length blond hair, but only Growing Up Skipper had the ability to transform herself "from a cute little girl to a tall curvy teenager" in seconds. This version of Barbie's little sister had an unusual way of going through puberty. When her left arm was rotated, her breasts grew, her waist shrank, and she got a little taller. When her arm was turned in the other direction, she became a kid again. Growing Up Skipper created a controversy when it was released in 1975; it was off the market two years later.

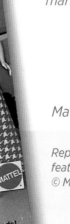

Mattel never made Growing Up Ken.

Reproduction of the 1961 original Ken doll featuring his famous red bathing suit.
© Mattel, Inc.

◗ I just turned 18. Is it still possible for my breasts to get bigger?

On average, most women are finished growing by age 18, although some might continue to grow into their early 20s. It is a good rule of thumb not to have breast surgery until your height, weight and breast size have been stable for two years.

◗ I was a small B in college; now I'm a C. Shouldn't I have stopped developing already?

Although you have probably finished developing, you may have gained weight. Breasts, which are made up mostly of fatty tissue, are often the first indicators of increased weight. In addition, birth control pills and pregnancy can increase your cup size, sometimes dramatically. Your breasts can even vary with each menstrual cycle. They may continue to change in size throughout your life.

◗ My mom has big breasts. Why don't I?

Breast size is determined primarily by heredity, and the genes responsible for it can come from a relative on either your mother's side or your father's side. Breast size also depends on hormone levels, whether or not you have been pregnant, and your percentage of body fat. That's why it is possible for your breasts to look nothing like your mother's or your sister's.

— Age 18

— Age 16

— Age 14

— Age 12

— Age 10

— Age 8

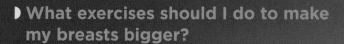

❱ What exercises should I do to make my breasts bigger?

Working out at the gym builds muscle, but there are no muscles in your breasts. That's why no number of chest presses, dumbbell flys or push-ups will pump 'em up. The breasts sit on top of the muscle and are made up predominantly of fatty tissue. You would have a better chance of increasing your breast size at the ice cream parlor.

◐◐ Titbit:
Unfortunately, an ice cream cone doesn't come with a GPS system to direct it to the chest instead of the thighs. Genetic predisposition determines where your excess fat is stored.

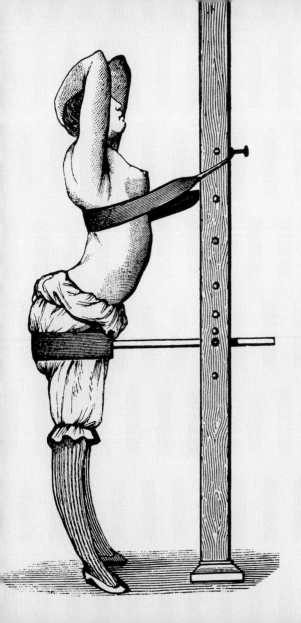

Gym Class Horrors

"We must, we must,
we must increase our bust.
The bigger the better,
the tighter the sweater,
The boys depend on us!"

In Judy Blume's 1970 novel, Are You There, God? It's Me, Margaret, *the main character and her sixth-grade classmates recite this chant while they do exercises to increase their breast size. Although the book is fiction, the chant is fact:*

In online forums, one man wrote, "I remember hearing girls doing that 'we must, we must' thing when I was in high school back in the 1950s; it was accompanied by some sort of exercise that was supposed to accomplish the 'increase our bust.'" One woman recalled her experience in the 1970s: "We had to do chest exercises in gym. This was extremely embarrassing, especially considering we had a male teacher. You placed the palms of your hands together and pressed them in rhythm to the chant."

19th century lady's fitness exerciser.

Can I increase my breast size by eating certain foods?

Soy products, pumpkin seeds, kidney beans, carrots and alfalfa sprouts are all estrogen-rich foods, but you couldn't eat enough of any of them to make your breasts grow. However, you could increase your breast size by eating a lot of high-fat junk food because your breasts will increase in size as the fat cells within them enlarge. So, too, will your hips, stomach and bottom, and not necessarily in that order.

Can I increase my breast size with herbs?

The all-natural herbal supplements formulated to enlarge your breasts sound exotic: American dwarf palm mixed with dong quai and blessed thistle; motherwort blended with dandelion root and wild yam. Herbs might help with digestion, lactation or menstrual cramps, but they won't grow your breasts – even if the manufacturer has thrown some phytoestrogen-rich plants into the mix.

In Search of Miracle-Gro

Phytoestrogens are estrogen-like chemicals that occur in a variety of plants. One source, Pueraria mirifica, is found in the forests of Thailand and Myanmar. Other sources include fenugreek (a spice common in the Middle East), ginseng, soybeans, carrots and berries.

(continued)

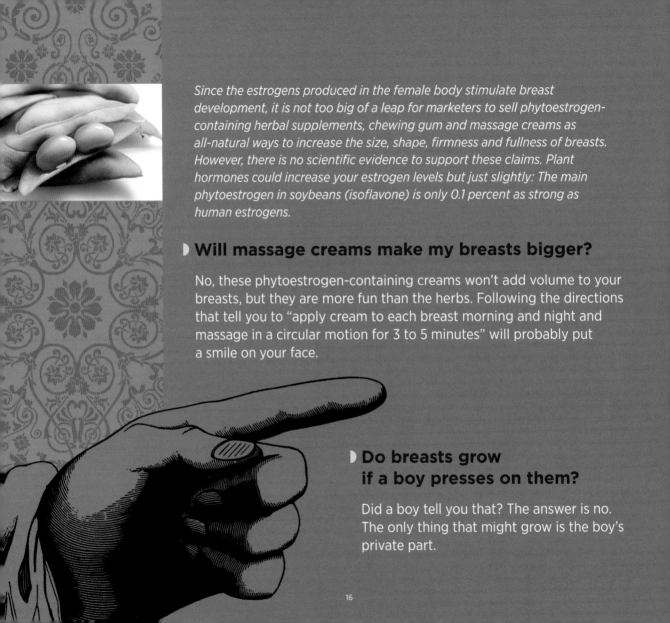

Since the estrogens produced in the female body stimulate breast development, it is not too big of a leap for marketers to sell phytoestrogen-containing herbal supplements, chewing gum and massage creams as all-natural ways to increase the size, shape, firmness and fullness of breasts. However, there is no scientific evidence to support these claims. Plant hormones could increase your estrogen levels but just slightly: The main phytoestrogen in soybeans (isoflavone) is only 0.1 percent as strong as human estrogens.

▶ Will massage creams make my breasts bigger?

No, these phytoestrogen-containing creams won't add volume to your breasts, but they are more fun than the herbs. Following the directions that tell you to "apply cream to each breast morning and night and massage in a circular motion for 3 to 5 minutes" will probably put a smile on your face.

▶ Do breasts grow if a boy presses on them?

Did a boy tell you that? The answer is no. The only thing that might grow is the boy's private part.

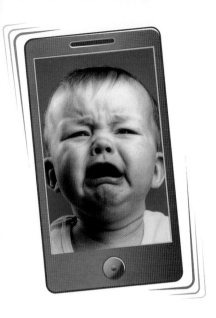

Who's Calling?

Japanese scientist Dr. Hideto Tomabechi has made it his mission to understand how sounds affect the brain and the body. So what did he do with his talents? He created "Rock Melon," a loud, scratchy-sounding cell phone ringtone that includes the subliminal cry of a baby. His theory is that the tone will cause a woman's brain to switch into motherhood mode, making her breasts fill with milk. After she hears it 20 times a day for 10 days in a row, her breasts will grow one inch; we suspect the noise will drive her insane first. And, as one skeptic asked, "If this works, shouldn't all women working in nurseries have huge breasts?"

What is the average breast size?

In much of the world, breast size has been increasing for the past two decades - from 36B to 36C in Europe and the United States, and from 34A to 34C across Asia. Men haven't wished this into being. It is related to the fact that we are getting fatter, too. As portion sizes grow, so do breasts. In 1999, researchers from the University of Newcastle reported that Australian women were 1 inch taller, 11 pounds heavier, and 1½ inches wider around the waist than their 1920's counterparts.

The Triumph International "Bra Usage and Attitude Study" of British women found that the average chest and hips measured 1½ inches more in 2010 than in the 1950s. One reporter conjectured that if the trend continues, the average British woman will be wearing somewhere between an F-cup and a G-cup bra in 50 years.

D-scribing British Women

A survey conducted by Triumph International, a manufacturer of intimate apparel, compared the percentage of women who wear A, B, C and D cup sizes in European countries. Results showed that British women have the biggest breasts (57 percent wear a D cup or larger) and Italian women the smallest breasts (68 percent wear a B cup).

Here is the list from biggest to smallest, in case you want to plan your next European vacation around it: United Kingdom, Denmark, Netherlands, Belgium, France, Sweden, Greece, Switzerland, Austria and Italy. We wonder when Calvin Klein will conduct a survey of men's underwear sizes.

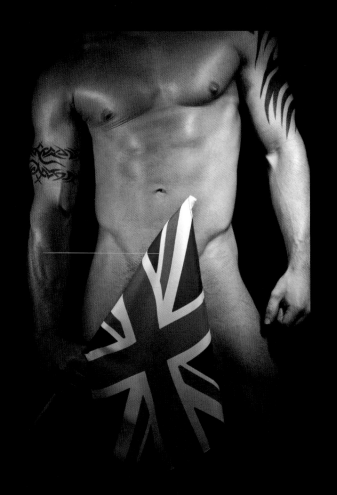

When will my breasts get saggy?

No crystal ball can predict how much and how soon your breasts will droop. Significant weight gain and then loss can cause the skin to stretch and the breasts to sag. So, too, can pregnancy, when the mammary glands produce milk and the breasts are temporarily enlarged.

As women age and hormone levels drop, the lobules (the part of the breast where milk is produced) shrink and breast volume is lost. At the same time, skin thins and loses its elasticity. You can observe this if you pinch (gently, please) the skin on your grandmother's hand. It will remain pinched longer than yours does.

How much does a breast weigh?

Breast weight is dependent on the size of the breast and the ratio of fatty tissue to dense tissue. To weigh your breast, you could immerse it in a bowl of water and measure how much water is displaced, or you could believe *The Times of India*, which reported that "the average breast weighs about 0.5 kilograms (1.1 pounds) and contributes to 4 to 5 percent of the body's total fat content." Unfortunately, the writer didn't define "average."

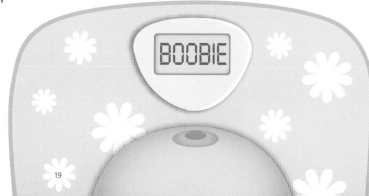

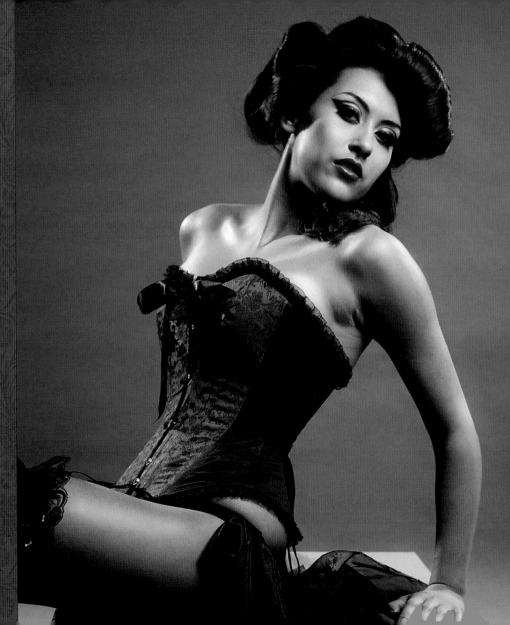

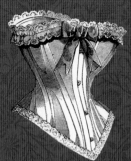

●●Titbit:
Cleavage was
fashionable in
Europe in the
1400s when bodices
and corsets were
designed to push
up the breasts.
Fast-forward 200
years to the court
of Louis XIV of
France, where
necklines were
lowered and
cleavage was
further exposed.
Cleavage was king,
so to speak, until
the 1920s when the
flat-chested flapper
look came into style.

Do I need big breasts to have cleavage?

No. Cleavage, or the intermammary sulcus (the less-sexy anatomical term), is the space between the breasts. Cleavage is delineated by where the fatty portion of each breast sits in relationship to the sternum, or breastbone. If your breasts are bigger, it is easier to push them together to accent the hollow between them.

When cleavage is enhanced with a push-up bra or exposed by a low-cut top, it draws a lot of attention. Scientists conjecture that the attraction to cleavage is primal: cleavage mimics the cleft between the buttocks, which we hide from view these days by wearing clothing and walking on two legs instead of four as our ancestors did.

Why aren't my breasts the same size?

Breasts are sisters, not twins. Few women have identical breasts; the difference might be slight or more obvious. Chances are one of your feet is slightly larger than the other one, too. That's because the two sides of the body are not perfectly matched mirror images. They are asymmetrical.

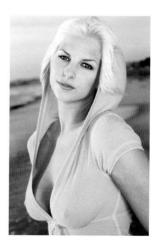

Nipple position, chest diameter, the amount of breast tissue, and the location of the breast on the chest wall all contribute to the appearance of your breasts. When one breast hangs a little lower than the other, it might give the illusion of being bigger. It might also look bigger when there is a longer distance from the nipple to the inframammary fold (the crease beneath the breast). With all these variables, it is no surprise that no one has identical twins.

(continued)

A severe but rare instance of asymmetry is Poland's syndrome, the absence and underdevelopment of the chest muscle on one side of the body. In girls, the breast on that side might never develop. In severe cases, Poland's syndrome can also affect the growth of the ribs and the arm. Both boys and girls can be born with the condition, but it is seen three times more frequently in boys.

▶ Does my left breast look a little bigger to you?

Maybe just a tiny bit, but join the crowd. It's recorded in the medical literature that the left breast is usually slightly larger than the right, and I've found this to be the case for about 9 out of every 10 of my patients.

No one knows for sure why the left breast is commonly bigger; some theorize that it is because the heart is on the left side. Others suggest that it is because right-handed women nurse their babies more often from their left breast, so they can keep their dominant hand free. (Ninety percent of the population is right-handed.)

What is a tubular breast?

A tubular breast is a breast that is long and narrow, like a tube sock, rather than the more common round shape. Often the breast is droopy and the areola is puffy. A tubular breast is considered a congenital defect; it first becomes visible at puberty when the mammary gland doesn't fully develop. Breast augmentation surgery will help improve the appearance of the breast itself, but it won't change the puffiness of the nipple. That can be improved by an areola reduction.

Why do some men have A or B cups?

It is not uncommon for an overweight man to have a buildup of fat deposits in his chest area, which may make it appear as if he has breasts. This is called pseudogynecomastia. Less commonly, men may have true gynecomastia, a hormonal imbalance (more estrogens than androgens) that causes the growth of glandular breast tissue. Some men choose to have surgery to remove the excess tissue.

⊙⊙Titbit: Infants and pubescent boys sometimes have short-term gynecomastia that disappears on its own in time.

THE MORE, THE MERRIER

Men seem to think that if two breasts are good, three are better, judging from the online admiration of the three-breasted mutant hooker who opened her blouse to entice Arnold Schwarzenegger in the 1990 sci-fi film Total Recall.

On the other hand, we have had a love-hate relationship with extra nipples throughout the centuries.

- **Love:** *In ancient times, extra nipples were considered a sign of increased fertility.*

- **Hate:** *In the 1690s in Salem, Massachusetts, a third nipple was the sign of a witch; women who had them were burned at the stake so they couldn't continue to suckle the devil.*

- **Hate:** *In the 1974 James Bond film* The Man With the Golden Gun, *the villain, Scaramanga, had a third nipple. Bond put on a fake nipple so he could impersonate his nemesis.*

- **Love:** *In 1995, actor Mark Wahlberg decided not to remove his third nipple, calling it his "prized possession."*

Fountain of Diana of Ephesus, Villa d'Este, Tivoli (Rome, Italy) features many breasts spewing out water.

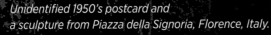

Unidentified 1950's postcard and a sculpture from Piazza della Signoria, Florence, Italy.

❱ Why do some women have extra nipples?

Extra nipples, known as supernumerary nipples or polythelia, are a fairly common congenital condition. The nipples usually show up along the milk ridge that runs from the armpit to the groin. They are often mistaken for moles since they tend to be small and not well-formed. These extra nipples are sometimes called "accessory nipples," but we don't think the woman with five nipples on her left breast and two on her right, described in a 1675 medical report, considered her accessory nipples a fashion statement.

When extra nipples appear with breast tissue and ducts, they are known as supernumerary breasts or polymastia. This rare condition might not show up until puberty. Extra breasts have been reported on the buttocks, face, upper arm and hip. A woman in Marseille, France, had an extra breast on the side of her left thigh. It produced milk when she was pregnant, and she used all three of her breasts to nurse her five children. In 1886, a doctor documented the case of a woman with 10 breasts, the highest number ever reported.

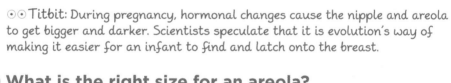

⊙⊙Titbit: During pregnancy, hormonal changes cause the nipple and areola to get bigger and darker. Scientists speculate that it is evolution's way of making it easier for an infant to find and latch onto the breast.

❱ What is the right size for an areola?

The judgment around size is personal and cultural. Areola size doesn't necessarily correspond to breast size. Some women have smaller breasts and larger areolas; others have larger breasts and smaller areolas. During breast reduction surgery, the areola is often reduced to 38 to 42 mm in width (about 1½ inches).

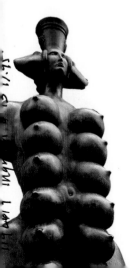

Cybele, the Goddess of Fertility, a sculpture by Mihail Chemiakin

What are the round bumps around my nipples?

They are Montgomery glands, and they were named for the Irish obstetrician who first identified them in the early 1800s. The glands secrete an oily fluid that keeps the nipples lubricated. During pregnancy, the glands often become more prominent.

Why does one of my nipples turn in instead of sticking out?

The tissue of your nipple is inverted (pulled in) rather than everted (pushed out). It is a normal variation – like having an "innie" instead of an "outie" belly button. Women sometimes ask if their nipple can be made into an "outie." Although a procedure can be done, it is not uncommon for the nipple to become inverted again.

⊙⊙ Titbit: One study reported that when erect, the typical female nipple is 8 mm, or 3/8 of an inch long. That's equal to about five stacked quarters.

POLITICALLY INCORRECT - *To help fund his 2010 election campaign to the Venezuelan National Assembly, Gustavo Rojas raffled off breast implants. "Raffle tickets ($6 each) on sale now: win a breast implant operation for yourself or your partner," he announced on his website. He wanted to unseat members of Hugo Chavez's United Socialist Party. The press had a field day, calling him a "political boob" who was "implanting democracy in Venezuela." He lost the election.*

One elementary school's AutoCorrect changed every reference to "boob" or "tit" to "breast." So guess what happened when a fifth grader typed "U.S. ConsTITution" into the school computer?
It changed it to ConsBREASTution.

POLITICAL BOOB

Vote Rojas

What's the Problem With Female Nipples?

On broadcast TV, websites, and in magazines, it's not uncommon to see women's nipples blurred or hidden behind black bars or stars. (Areolas are outlawed, too.) And when a celebrity has a "nip slip," the censors go crazy and the fans go to TheNipSlip.com.

Citing its no-pornography policy, Facebook has removed photos of a mother breastfeeding her infant and of a naked porcelain doll (with nipples) that was part of a jewelry ad. Because of Apple's no-nipple policy, fashion magazines have to censor ads and photo spreads in their iPad editions.

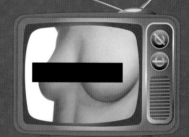

What's up with the no-female-nipple policy? Why do they allow photos of cleavage but not nipples? Why don't they censor men's nipples? Is it because, as Ms. Magazine *blogger Lisa Wade wrote, "Men have chests and women have breasts"? This double standard rests on a "jiggly foundation," she quipped.*

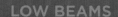

LOW BEAMS

In the 1920s, burlesque dancers and strippers used pasties (nipple covers) to cover up their nipples so they didn't get arrested for performing topless. These days, women use them when they want a little coverage but can't, or don't want to, wear a bra. So it's no surprise that nipple covers, from companies like Nippies, Smooth'em and Low Beams, are a big business. There are hundreds to choose from in silicone, satin and faux leather: disposable or reusable; hearts, stars or circles; leopard prints, gold lamé or nude.

Coffee or Tea?

The first bras had stretchable cups that were supposed to accommodate breasts of various sizes, but one size did not fit all. So in the 1930s, manufacturers introduced bras with a range of cup sizes.

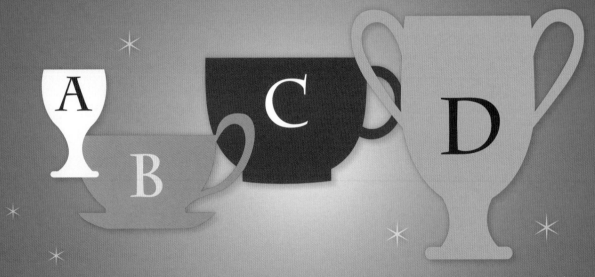

While British bra makers used discreet descriptions like "junior" and "medium," American companies were more upfront. The Formfit Company offered "small," "average" and "full" cup sizes in each band. A few years later, Warner's introduced its "Alphabet Bra" with A, B, C and D cups. Before too long, these cup sizes got nicknames: egg cup, tea cup, coffee cup and challenge cup.

A shop assistant for the Spirella corset company described a different classification system: "The 'Totalitarian' is designed for suppression of the masses, the 'Salvation Army' to uplift the fallen, and the 'Political Agitator' to make mountains out of molehills." – Spirella company newsletter, Jan. 1959

GO AHEAD AND TITTER

If you say "tit" on broadcast television, it will probably get bleeped, but these "tit"-containing words will get past the censors:

- **tit for tat** - *getting even; equal retaliation; an eye for an eye*

- **Titicaca** - *the highest lake in the world, located in the Andes Mountains on the border between Peru and Bolivia*

- **titillate** - *to excite or arouse*

- **titivate** - *to make yourself look attractive, perhaps by putting on makeup or doing your hair*

- **titman** - *the runt of a litter, especially the smallest pig*

- **titmouse** - *a small North American songbird*

- **titter** - *a restrained, half-suppressed laugh; a giggle*

- **tittle** - *a tiny amount or part of something*

- **tittle-tattle** - *idle talk; gossip*

- **titubation** - *a nodding movement of the head or body; a tremor, commonly caused by a nervous disorder*

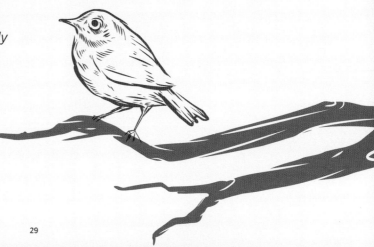

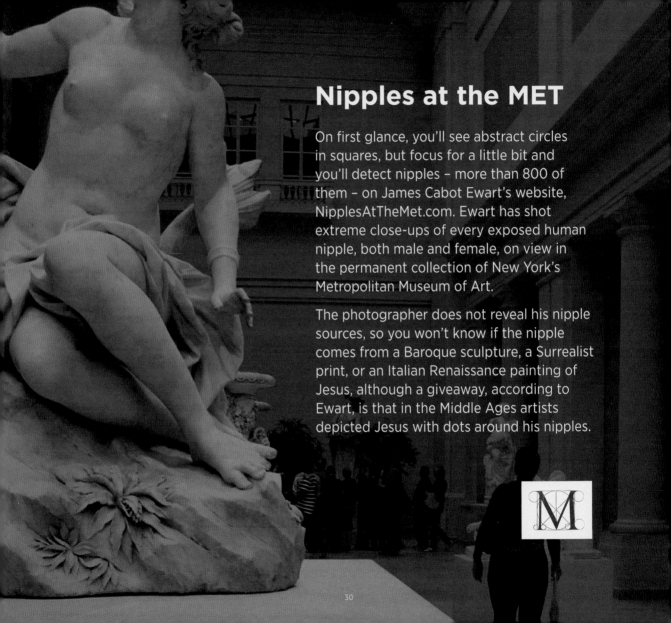

Nipples at the MET

On first glance, you'll see abstract circles in squares, but focus for a little bit and you'll detect nipples – more than 800 of them – on James Cabot Ewart's website, NipplesAtTheMet.com. Ewart has shot extreme close-ups of every exposed human nipple, both male and female, on view in the permanent collection of New York's Metropolitan Museum of Art.

The photographer does not reveal his nipple sources, so you won't know if the nipple comes from a Baroque sculpture, a Surrealist print, or an Italian Renaissance painting of Jesus, although a giveaway, according to Ewart, is that in the Middle Ages artists depicted Jesus with dots around his nipples.

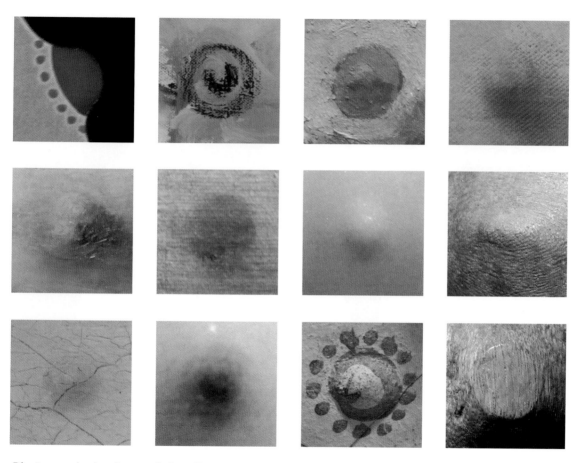

Photographs by James Cabot Ewart

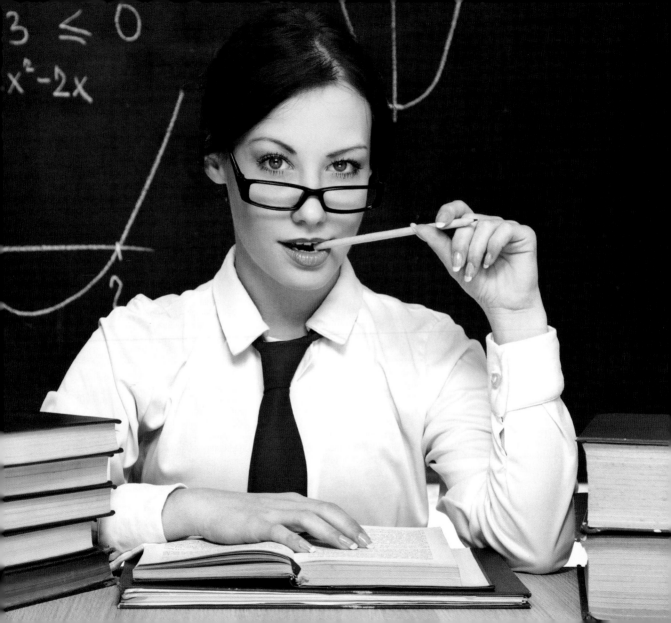

Chapter 2

The ABCs of Double Ds

Will my implants help me float? Could I take them on a boat?
Could I bring them on a plane? What will happen in the rain?
If I squeeze them will they pop? Will I fit in my old top?
In the sauna will they boil? Are they filled with cooking oil?
Will they freeze up in the cold? Will they droop down when I'm old?
Can I get them if I'm high? What will happen when I die?

– Inspired by "Green Eggs and Ham"
by Dr. Seuss

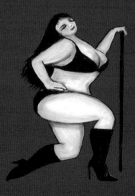

◗ What implants are approved for use in the United States?

The U.S. Food and Drug Administration (FDA) recognizes three implant manufacturers (Allergan, Mentor and Sientra) and two types of implants (saline and silicone gel). Each comes in a variety of sizes, shapes, profiles and textures.

◗ Why were silicone gel implants unavailable for so many years?

In December 1990, CBS-TV reporter Connie Chung hosted a show on the alleged dangers of silicone gel breast implants; she interviewed women who believed that their ruptured implants caused breast cancer and a range of autoimmune diseases.

In 1992, the FDA determined that manufacturers had not provided adequate information "to demonstrate that silicone gel breast implants were safe and effective."

IMPLANTS	SALINE	SILICONE GEL
Shell	silicone	silicone
Filler	sterile saline (salt water)	silicone gel
Size range (moderate profile)	125-775 cubic centimeters (ccs)	100-800 ccs
Filling	inserted empty and then filled	prefilled
Incision	approx. 1½ inches	approx. 2 inches
Minimum age	18	22

The agency removed them from the market with a few exceptions: They could still be used for reconstruction after mastectomy, to correct congenital deformities, and to replace existing silicone gel breast implants. Women were enrolled in clinical trials so that data could be collected about the safety of these implants.

In 2006, after reviewing the data and failing to find a link between silicone gel breast implants and disease, the FDA lifted its 14-year restriction and approved them for all women 22 and older.

Should I get teardrop implants?

Implants come in two shapes – round and teardrop (also called anatomic). If you were interested in mostly lower breast fullness, teardrop implants would be appropriate. However, the large majority of women express interest in upper breast fullness, which is better accomplished with round implants.

How do I know what implant profile to ask for?

Profile refers to an implant's width and forward projection; the narrower the implant, the more it projects. The implant profile is selected according to the width of your breast, which will be measured during your consultation. If you have a larger frame and wider breasts, lower- or medium-profile implants will better conform to your shape. If you have a small frame, you might be a candidate for higher-profile implants, the narrowest of all.

Overs and Unders: Implant Placement

Subglandular placement refers to implants placed behind the breast but in front of – or over – the pectoral muscle. Submuscular placement refers to implants placed behind – or under – that muscle. In general, I prefer to put implants behind the muscle because I believe they look more natural. Also, there may be less chance of infection and capsular contraction (hardness) and less interference during a mammogram (X-ray of the breast).

Do silicone gel implants feel more natural?

It depends on their placement. When you hold a saline implant in one hand and a silicone gel implant in the other, the silicone gel implant feels softer. Likewise, when the implants are placed in front of the pectoral muscle and are covered only by your breast tissue, silicone gel implants feel more natural.

When they are placed behind the muscle, saline and silicone gel implants feel similar in most women. The exception is in very slender women who have thin skin, less breast tissue, and little or no muscle coverage around the side and underneath their breasts – the areas where the implant could most likely be felt. If this were a concern for you, silicone gel implants would be a better option.

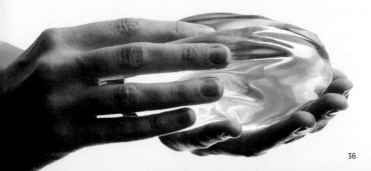

Can I get "gummy bear" implants?

Not if you live in the United States. "Gummy bears" is the nickname for a highly cohesive silicone gel breast implant that resembles the candy; the gel is semisolid and holds its shape. Although "gummy bears" have been used around the world for about 15 years, they are still being tested in the United States. At the present time, they are available only to patients enrolled in clinical trials. The silicone gel breast implants available in the United States are made of cohesive silicone gel, too, but it is a softer semisolid that changes shape as you move. "Cohesive" means that the silicone gel is unlikely to leak if the implant shell tears.

What's That Smell?

Soybean oil is a good source of vitamin E and omega-3 fatty acids. The oil might even strengthen your nails, but it is not an ideal filler for breast implants. That's what a British company learned in 1995 when it marketed Trilucent breast implants filled with medical-grade triglycerides extracted from soybean oil. When the oil leaked, some women had a local reaction that included pain and swelling. Others reported that their breasts had a foul odor. Turns out the oil had gone rancid. Masking that smell is a tall order for even the best deodorant. The implants were taken off the market just four years after their introduction.

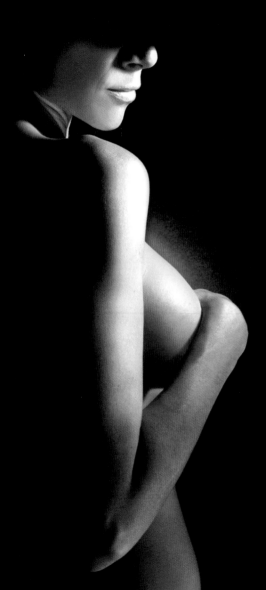

Can my implants grow inside of me?

Only if they are "string implants," which are banned in the United States and the European Union. String implants are made from polypropylene, a fiberlike material that, when implanted, irritates the breast pocket. The irritation produces fluid, which is absorbed by the implants, and the implants expand into abnormally large, cartoonish breasts. There are reports of each breast reaching a weight of 25 pounds or more, and because the material is unpredictable, the implants can grow at different rates.

Do breast implants glow in the dark?

If you shine a flashlight underneath or next to your augmented breasts, they will cast an eerie glow. It's a great party trick. The narrator of the "Glowing Boobs" YouTube video says, "They are the most joyful, wonderful glow sticks you can ever imagine ... which last much longer than regular glow sticks and you never have to put them in the freezer." In case you were wondering, saline implants glow a little brighter than silicone gel implants.

Do implants cause breast cancer?

There are no conclusive studies to indicate that breast implants are unsafe. On its website, the American Cancer Society states, "Silicone breast implants can cause scar tissue to form in the breast. But studies have found that this does not increase breast cancer risk." The FDA, implant manufacturers, and scientists continue to research and evaluate the safety of breast implants.

Do implants get in the way of reading a mammogram?

More than one-third of a million women have breast augmentation surgery each year, which means that radiologists are likely to have experience evaluating breasts with implants. When you schedule your mammogram, it's important to let the facility know that you have breast implants. To maximize the amount of breast tissue that can be seen, the technician will gently displace (push up) the implants and will take extra views of each breast.

In a small percentage of cases, implants cast a shadow on breast tissue and partially obscure the view, making it more difficult for the radiologist to detect an abnormality. When implants are placed behind the muscle, there is less shadow cast and less chance of interference.

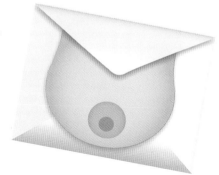

"Whoever thought up the word 'mammogram'? Every time I hear it, I think I'm supposed to put my breast in an envelope and send it to someone."

– Jan King, Medicine Ball vocalist and guitarist

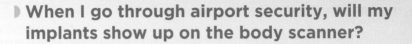

When I go through airport security, will my implants show up on the body scanner?

A full-body scanner produces X-ray images, and it is very likely that your implants will show up. However, the Transportation Security Administration (TSA) inspector will be in another room viewing the pictures on a monitor and should not be broadcasting the news. One way to keep your breast augmentation surgery private is to refuse the scan and request a pat-down instead. You have the legal right to do so. It's highly unlikely that the TSA agent will be able to feel your breast implants.

Another Definition of Bombshell

After a Nigerian man tried to blow up a plane with explosives packed into his underpants, British intelligence agents reportedly picked up chatter from Pakistan and Yemen that warned them about another disturbing possibility: Female suicide bombers recruited by al-Qaeda may have gotten breast implants packed with an explosive known as PETN. Five ounces would be enough to blow a hole in a jumbo jet. The new body scanners probably wouldn't have detected the explosives; critics say the technology is useful for detecting guns and knives but ineffective against thin plastics, gels and liquids.

⊙⊙ Titbit: By government regulation, standard in-flight cabin pressure is equivalent to what you would experience at about 8,000 feet – the altitude of Vail, Colorado.

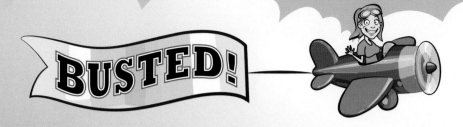

Is it true that my implants will explode at 35,000 feet?

No, but it didn't stop Spike TV from saying so. An episode of *1000 Ways to Die*, titled "Titty Titty, Bang Bang," showed a woman who exploded on a flight to Vegas when the liquid in her implants expanded. If this were true, wouldn't many Hollywood actresses have exploded by now?

MythBusters, a more scientifically sound television program, had busted that myth years earlier. Their research team put implants in a hypobaric chamber, recreated the altitude at 35,000 feet, and observed that the implants expanded insignificantly. Other researchers took breast implants on a simulated trip from the bottom of the ocean to the top of Mount Everest, and the implants still didn't burst. This means that if you went to 35,000 feet in an unpressurized airplane, your implants would be safe. Unfortunately, you would be dead in about 10 minutes from hypoxia (oxygen deficiency).

Pack 'Em in Your Luggage

The TSA says that liquids and gels are safe to bring aboard an aircraft in limited amounts – 3.4 ounces or less. Thank goodness your implants are "packed in your luggage," so to speak, because one 425 cc implant is equal to about 14 ounces. It would be hard to squeeze it into one of those quart-sized plastic bags. To figure out how many ounces your implants are, divide the number of cubic centimeters in each of them by 30.

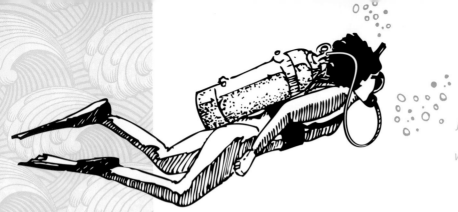

▶ Will scuba diving harm my breast implants?

No. A research team at Duke University Medical Center placed silicone gel and saline implants in a hyperbaric chamber to simulate the pressure experienced by scuba divers at various depths. When a diver is underwater, the increased pressure causes nitrogen, a component of the air we breathe, to build up in the blood and body tissues. If a diver surfaces too quickly, the nitrogen gas can form dangerous bubbles, similar to the bubbles you see when you first open a bottle of soda.

So what happened to the breast implants? The medical experts at DAN, the Divers Alert Network, summarized the findings on their website: "The bubbles that formed in the implants led to a small volume increase, which is not likely to damage the implants or surrounding tissues. If gas bubbles do form in the implant, they resolve over time."

P.S. No implants were harmed in the study.

Will breast implants keep me afloat in the ocean?

No. Here's why: Most people are neutrally buoyant, which means they don't float up or down; they hover. More fat makes you float; more muscle makes you sink. It is gravity that eventually pulls you down.

Saline implants are filled with salt water in about the same density as the ocean water you are swimming in, so they are neutrally buoyant, too. You will float more easily in the ocean than in a pool because salt water is heavier than fresh water, but the same basic principles apply.

Silicone gel implants are slightly denser than water. Although they won't make you sink, you might have to doggie paddle just a little bit harder. That's why it is recommended that after getting silicone gel implants, a scuba diver does a checkout dive to see if she needs to adjust her dive weights.

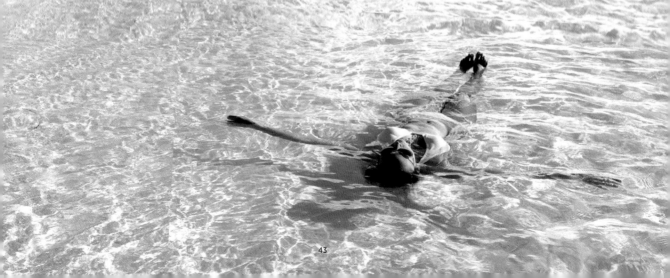

Bulgaria – A 24-year-old woman driver survived a head-on crash, thanks to her 40DD silicone-augmented breasts. A police expert explained: "The implants worked just like airbags – protecting the victim's ribs and vital organs from damage."

California – A 41-year-old dental receptionist who was shot in the chest with a semiautomatic assault rifle survived because her size-D breast implants absorbed much of the bullet's impact. According to her cosmetic surgeon, "The bullet fragments were millimeters from her heart and her vital organs. If she didn't have implants, she might not be alive today."

Jerusalem – A 24-year-old Israeli woman was wounded in a Hezbollah rocket attack. Doctors at Nahariya Hospital in northern Israel found shrapnel embedded in her silicone gel implants, just inches from her heart. A hospital spokesman said her breast implants "saved her from death."

P.S. None of the implants survived.

Will my breast implants freeze up in really cold weather?

Because your breast implants are close to your body, your natural body heat will keep them warm. As one blogger wrote, "Even if theoretically the girl was like a reptile or something and had no body heat, the freezing point of the material used in the implants would be pretty low." In other words, your implants could freeze, but before they did, you would die of hypothermia (dangerously low body temperature).

Will my breast implants be colder than the rest of my body?

Implants change temperature very slowly. If you swim in a cold pool or skate at an ice rink, your implants could cool to slightly below your body temperature, and they could feel cool to the touch. Likewise, if you hang out in a hot tub or spend the day sunbathing at the beach, your implants could feel warm to the touch. Implants that are placed behind the pectoral muscle are less susceptible to temperature changes.

⊙⊙Titbit: Outside of the body, a saline implant would freeze at about 28 degrees Fahrenheit, while a silicone gel implant would ice up at around 170 below zero.

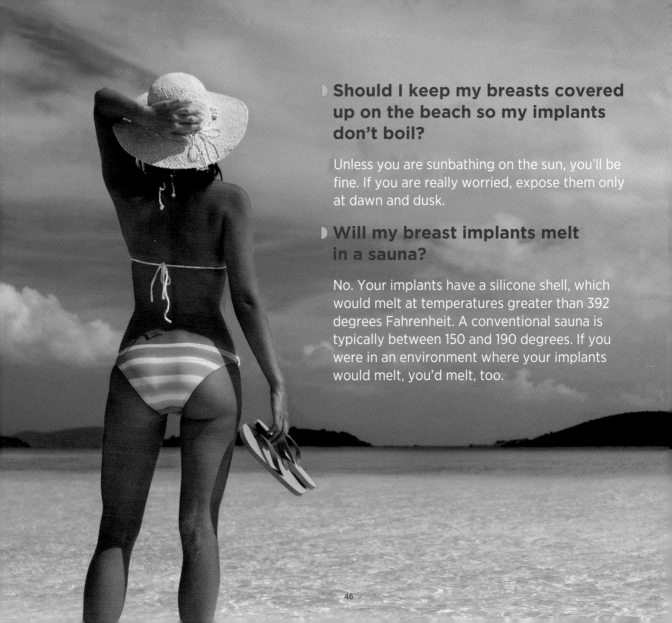

Should I keep my breasts covered up on the beach so my implants don't boil?

Unless you are sunbathing on the sun, you'll be fine. If you are really worried, expose them only at dawn and dusk.

Will my breast implants melt in a sauna?

No. Your implants have a silicone shell, which would melt at temperatures greater than 392 degrees Fahrenheit. A conventional sauna is typically between 150 and 190 degrees. If you were in an environment where your implants would melt, you'd melt, too.

Will an infrared sauna ruin my implants?

No. An infrared sauna is not as hot as a conventional sauna. An infrared sauna heats you through a process called conversion. It emits radiant heat that is absorbed directly into your body and has little effect on the temperature of the surrounding air. By contrast, a conventional sauna heats you indirectly: it warms the air, which in turn warms you.

Will my implants cook in a tanning bed?

Tanning salons use ultraviolet rays, which don't cook anything. They don't use microwaves, even though some people think they do. That was proved by a 2005 episode of *MythBusters*, when the crew placed two raw chickens in a tanning bed for one hour. The skin got a little darker, but the chickens were still raw inside.

Will my implants boil in a hot tub?

No. Your implants are inside of your body, and you would have to boil the outside of your body before the inside boiled. The average hot tub temperature of 102 degrees Fahrenheit isn't hot enough to do that.

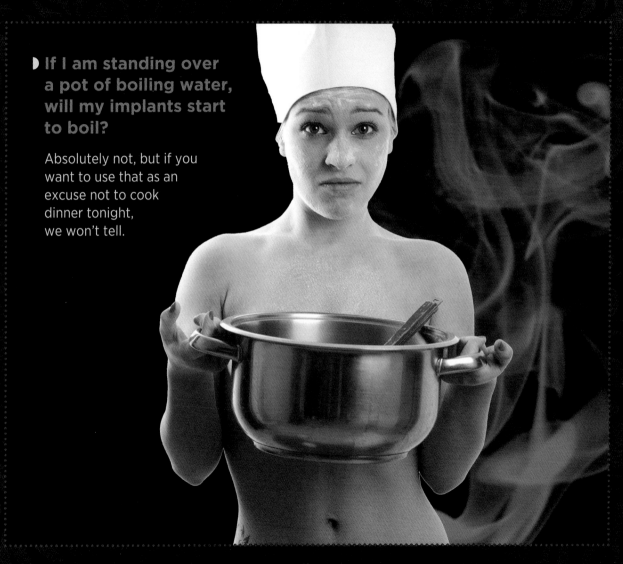

If I am standing over a pot of boiling water, will my implants start to boil?

Absolutely not, but if you want to use that as an excuse not to cook dinner tonight, we won't tell.

Will a mammogram pop my breast implants?

Breast implants are designed to be sturdy, and each manufacturer has its own testing protocol. Allergan tests its implants by exerting nearly 55 pounds of force on them repeatedly, up to 6.5 million times. By contrast, a routine mammogram exerts about 40 pounds of force when it compresses the breast, and if a woman had 50 mammograms in her lifetime, it would be a lot.

Can extreme mental stress cause breast implants to rupture?

Stress can affect every system of your body, from respiratory (shortness of breath) to reproductive (a shortened or lengthened menstrual cycle), but it cannot create enough force to make your breast implants break.

Let's imagine that you fell into a trash compactor. That would cause extreme mental stress and your implants could break, but it is the force of the compactor that would cause the damage – not the stress of the situation. So my advice is: Don't jump to conclusions or fall into a trash compactor.

IN NEED OF STRESS RELIEF?

How about squeezing a stress ball? They are made of gel or foam and are not necessarily round. Some light up; others laugh. They are shaped like brains or baseballs or breasts. You're not surprised, are you? You can even imprint your company logo on them and give them away at the next Christmas party.

When a regular-sized boob stress ball just won't do: The Giant Boob Stress Ball is available from www.find-me-a-gift.co.uk.

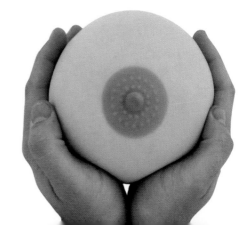

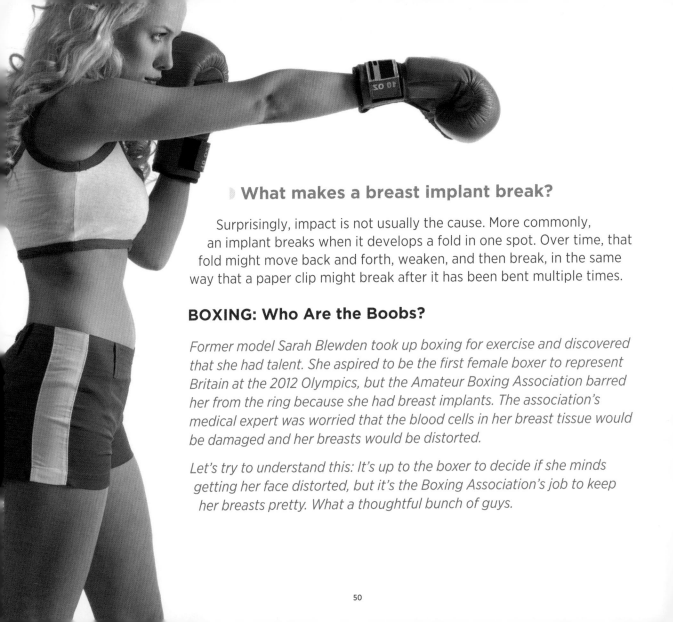

❱ What makes a breast implant break?

Surprisingly, impact is not usually the cause. More commonly, an implant breaks when it develops a fold in one spot. Over time, that fold might move back and forth, weaken, and then break, in the same way that a paper clip might break after it has been bent multiple times.

BOXING: Who Are the Boobs?

Former model Sarah Blewden took up boxing for exercise and discovered that she had talent. She aspired to be the first female boxer to represent Britain at the 2012 Olympics, but the Amateur Boxing Association barred her from the ring because she had breast implants. The association's medical expert was worried that the blood cells in her breast tissue would be damaged and her breasts would be distorted.

Let's try to understand this: It's up to the boxer to decide if she minds getting her face distorted, but it's the Boxing Association's job to keep her breasts pretty. What a thoughtful bunch of guys.

▶ Do breast implants need to be replaced every 10 years?

No. Your breast implants don't have an expiration date. Unlike your car, there is no maintenance required. You don't have to check the fluid levels regularly, and there's no need for a front-end alignment after 10,000 miles. Implants need to be replaced only if they break, and they are not that fragile. Through the years, manufacturers have increased the strength of the implant shell; in my experience, only about 3 percent of implants break. I had a patient who wanted to go bigger after 15 years. When I removed her implants, they looked exactly as they did the day I put them in.

▶ Will my breast implants get hard after a while?

The implant itself doesn't change or harden, but the newly formed lining (the capsule) around the implant could shrink and thicken, limiting the space in which the implant moves and making it feel hard. This is called capsular contraction. No one knows the exact cause, but theories include infection, bleeding and trauma, all of which are rare. Only two of my 5,000 patients have had capsular contraction.

⊙⊙Titbit: Imagine that you are blowing a bubblegum bubble. It is round and thin. That thin gum is similar to the normal lining that starts to form around breast implants as early as three weeks after surgery. When the bubble breaks, the gum shrinks and thickens, much like the lining around the implant does when there is capsular contraction. This shrunken lining is often referred to as scar tissue.

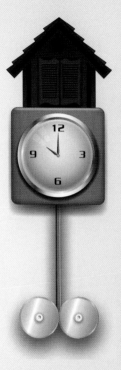

Can I be identified by my breast implants if something happens to me?

Each saline and silicone gel breast implant is assigned a lot number and a serial number, but only the lot number is laser engraved on the implant. The 2009 news report about a murdered woman who was identified by her breast implants is misleading; although police were able to read the lot number, size and style imprinted on her implants, they had to do further detective work to establish her identity.

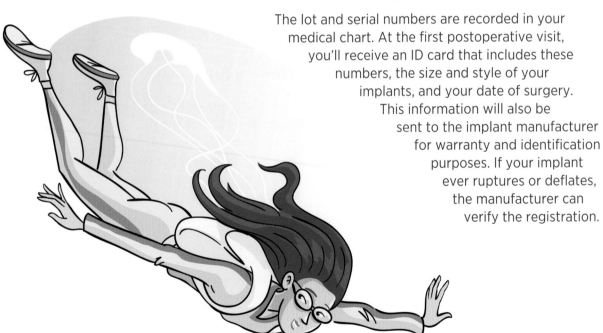

The lot and serial numbers are recorded in your medical chart. At the first postoperative visit, you'll receive an ID card that includes these numbers, the size and style of your implants, and your date of surgery. This information will also be sent to the implant manufacturer for warranty and identification purposes. If your implant ever ruptures or deflates, the manufacturer can verify the registration.

▶ What happens to my breast implants when I die?

They are left just as they are. Funeral homes don't remove breast implants, artificial joints, surgical staples, or artificial heart valves. And unlike the rest of you, your implants will not decompose. They have a shell of medical grade silicone, which falls into the class of inert, inorganic rubbers.

The only exception is when an autopsy is performed. In that case, according to one funeral home director, "an incision is made from the shoulder to the nipple, and implants are removed. The implants come back whole in a plastic bag."

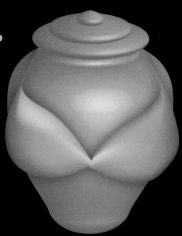

▶ Do breast implants have to be removed before cremation?

No. Although the new silicone bakeware won't burn up in an oven, your implants will. That's because a crematorium is between 1,600 and 1,800 degrees Fahrenheit. However, in her "Funky Facts About Cremation" blog post, horror writer Deborah LeBlanc warns, "The cremains can stick to the residual silicone, which means you'll wind up with clumps of Aunt Erma instead of gritty ash."

Bosom Buddies

When her husband died in a car accident, a young Australian woman allegedly had his cremated remains sewn into her breast implants so she could keep him close to her heart. The news generated a lot of online comments, such as, "Now his relatives will always look at her boobs and cry," and "I wonder if that would be a good excuse to cop a feel and say: 'I just want to pay respects to my dear brother.'"

Look Familiar?

Mushrooms and melons and mountains, oh my...

You don't have to look too hard to find "things that look like boobs but aren't," as one website puts it. Some are shaped by human hands, like cream puffs and the thatched-roof huts of Papua, New Guinea. Others are creations of nature, like acorns and Wyoming's Grand Tetons (French for "large teats").

Thank you, Mother Nature.

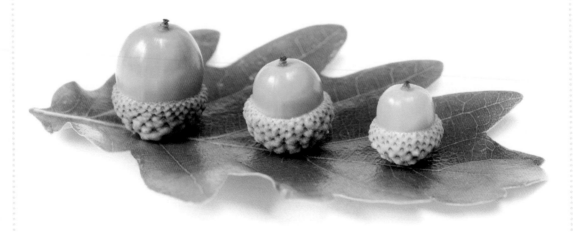

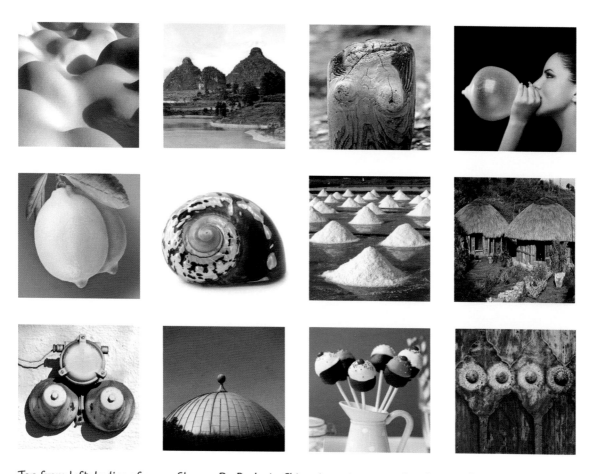

Top from left: bodies of snow, Shuang Ru Peaks in China, tree stump, condom being inflated.
Center from left: lemons, conch shell, sea salt field, Papua New Guinea grass huts.
Bottom from left: old doorbells, Playfair Observatory dome, cake pops, antique wooden door.

A BUSTLINE TIMELINE

1889: Austrian surgeon Robert Gersuny experiments by injecting paraffin wax into breasts, which get lumpy, hard and infected. During this period, breasts are also stuffed with glass balls, ground rubber, ivory, wool and ox cartilage.

1895: Czech surgeon Vincenz Czerny performs the first modern breast reconstruction. He removes a large noncancerous tumor from a woman's breast; before closing the wound, he implants a fist-sized lipoma (a benign tumor of fatty tissue) that he had removed from her back.

1920: Doctors attempt to enlarge breasts with fatty tissue taken from the stomach and buttocks. The body absorbs the fat over time, and the breasts get lumpy and uneven. The approach is abandoned in 1940.

1930s: Dow Corning develops silicone for use as an insulator, coolant and lubricant.

1940s: During World War II, hoping to attract American soldiers, Japanese prostitutes inject their breasts with liquid silicone. Direct injections are also widely used by Las Vegas showgirls. By the late 1960s, the practice is abandoned because of serious complications.

1950s: Doctors insert synthetic sponges into the breast, but the sponges shrink and harden within a year.

1961: Texas plastic surgeons Frank Gerow and Thomas Cronin insert silicone gel into an inert silicone shell to make silicone breast implants. They got the idea when they felt the new plastic bags that were being used for blood collection.

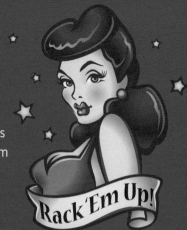

1962: Timmie Jean Lindsey of Texas becomes the first woman to receive silicone gel breast implants.

1963: Dow Corning begins marketing silicone gel implants under the trade name Silastic and is the only supplier until 1968.

1965: Plastic Surgeon H.G. Arion produces saline breast implants in France. He holds the copyright for the world's first inflatable prosthesis.

1968: Other companies enter the market by creating their own implant shells, but they have to depend on Dow Corning for the silicone gel to fill them.

1976: Congress passes the Medical Device Amendments to the Federal Food, Drug and Cosmetic Act, making breast implants subject to government regulation for the first time.

1992: The FDA creates a voluntary moratorium on silicone gel breast implants, requesting that manufacturers stop supplying them and surgeons stop implanting them. During the suspension, the FDA plans to review new information about the implants' safety and effectiveness.

2003: The FDA gives saline-filled implants its official stamp of approval for women who are at least 18 years old.

2006: After studies fail to find a link between silicone gel implants and disease, the FDA lifts its 14-year ban and approves silicone gel implants for women 22 and older.

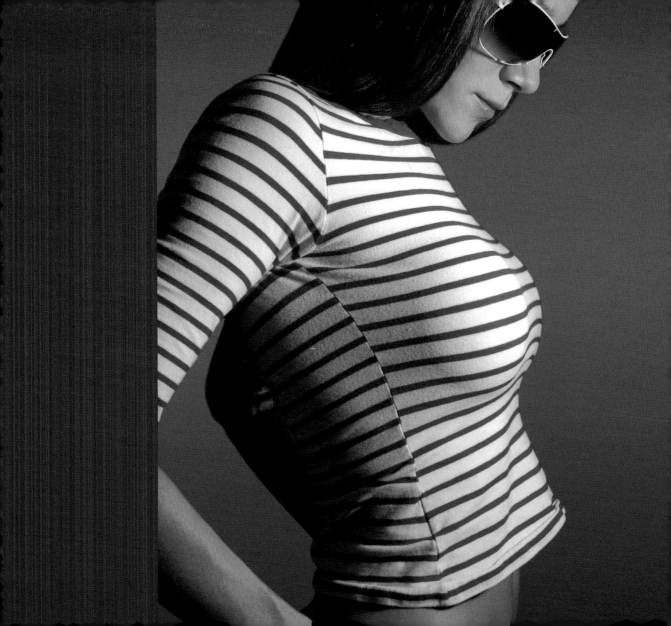

Chapter 3

To B or Not to B
a C or a D

Each year, more than 300,000 women in the United States
have breast augmentation surgery,
making it the No. 1 cosmetic surgery procedure.

For these women, the road from "thinking about it" to "doing it"
is paved with many questions and answers, like these ...

Foxy (Great-Grand) Mama

Cosmetic surgery is on the rise among older Americans, according to the American Society for Aesthetic Plastic Surgery, which reported that in 2011 close to 100,000 people age 65 and older had elective surgical procedures. While the majority had facelifts and cosmetic eyelid surgery, about 11,000 had cosmetic breast surgery. Among these was an 83-year-old great-grandmother from California who got a breast lift and implants.

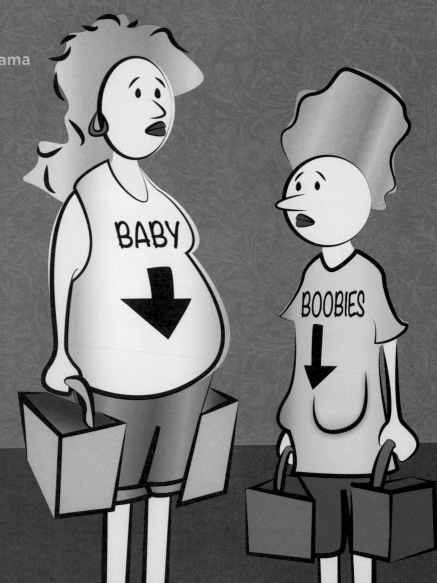

AM I A CANDIDATE?

⟩ Do I need a breast augmentation?

No one needs a breast augmentation. If you were to come into my office and ask me what I think you should do, I would ask you what you want. It would be very arrogant of me to tell you what to do. Plus, after taking care of more than 5,000 women – and being married for a long time – it's clear to me that women know what they want and that my job is just to listen.

But if you think an augmentation might make a difference for you, we would continue the consultation to find a match between your expectations and what I could accomplish surgically.

⟩ I'm turning 52 next week. Am I too old for implants?

Absolutely not. There's nothing wrong with wanting to look as good on the outside as you feel on the inside, no matter how old you are. If breast implants would make you feel better about how you look – in clothes or out – there's no reason to rule out cosmetic breast surgery.

To date, my oldest patient was 63. She had small breasts and had been thinking about getting implants for a long time. She had a new boyfriend, and the time was right for her. What's most important is that she was in good health.

Beauty Pageants

With Them . . .

If you've got them, want to flaunt them, are at least 18 and live in Hungary, you could compete in the next Miss Plastic Hungary Pageant. But first, you will have to submit your medical records to prove that you have been surgically enhanced. The grand-prize winner receives a brand new apartment, and her plastic surgeon wins a prize for his or her handiwork.

In past years, nearly all the contestants showed off augmented breasts. Reshaped noses were popular; just one finalist had surgically adjusted toes. Contestants were supposed to show a "perfect harmony of body and soul," but there were no pageant interviews during which the women could express their wishes for world peace.

. . . and Without Them

The tiny town of Isafjordur, Iceland, hosted an alternative beauty contest to celebrate body imperfections. Droopy breasts, cellulite, wrinkles and hairy backs were all considered signs of character and sex appeal. The only requirement: No plastic surgery. The pageant was open to men and women age 20 and over.

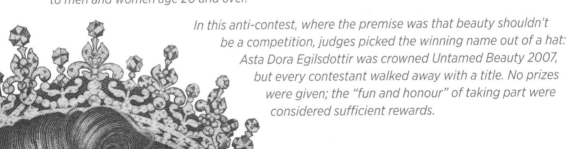

In this anti-contest, where the premise was that beauty shouldn't be a competition, judges picked the winning name out of a hat: Asta Dora Egilsdottir was crowned Untamed Beauty 2007, but every contestant walked away with a title. No prizes were given; the "fun and honour" of taking part were considered sufficient rewards.

▷ I just turned 18. Am I too young to get implants?

You are not too young to get saline implants, according to guidelines from the FDA and implant manufacturers, but you are not eligible for silicone gel implants until you are 22.

Age isn't the only deciding factor. You also need to be fully grown before you have cosmetic breast surgery, which means that there have been no changes in your height, weight or breast size for two years. Although most women finish growing by age 18, others continue to grow into their early 20s. You also need to have the emotional maturity to cope with the body image changes that result from cosmetic breast surgery.

▷ Can I get implants for my Sweet 16?

In the last decade, there was an increase in the number of teens who had breast augmentation surgery at age 16, despite FDA recommendations against it. While some doctors may take care of patients who are younger than 18, I do not.

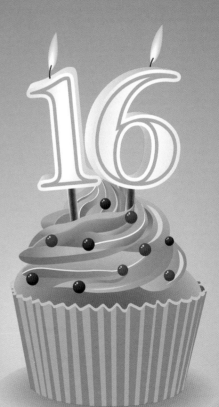

I'm on a diet. Should I finish losing weight before I get implants?

When you lose weight, it not only reduces the size of your waist and thighs, but it might also reduce the size of your breasts – sometimes dramatically. If this happens, you might be left with saggy breasts and stretched skin.

If you are planning to lose 10 percent or more of your body weight, it makes sense to wait until you have reached your goal before you have breast augmentation surgery. In order to choose breast implants that will make you proportional, you need to know your true starting size.

☉☉Titbit: If you are dieting, be sure to save a few dollars for shoe shopping. Some women report that along with losing a cup size, they lose a shoe size.

I'm hoping to get pregnant in the next year. Should I wait to have surgery?

If you are thinking about having a child in the next year or working on it now, I would suggest that you wait because your post-pregnancy breasts might look different from your current pair.

During pregnancy, your breasts will enlarge from hormonal changes and milk production. Afterward, they might return to their original size or get smaller, bigger or droopier. You won't know the verdict until six months after you have stopped breastfeeding or, if you are not breastfeeding, six months after childbirth.

If parenthood is further in your future and you are anxious to enjoy new breasts now, you don't have to wait. Just understand that you might need a revision after pregnancy.

◗ Will I be able to breastfeed after I get breast implants?

In most cases, breast augmentation surgery will not interfere with breastfeeding because milk ducts are generally not disturbed during the procedure. When implants are placed through an incision made around the areola, milk ducts are sometimes disrupted, which may affect breastfeeding. However, not all women are naturally able to breastfeed, whether or not they have cosmetic breast surgery.

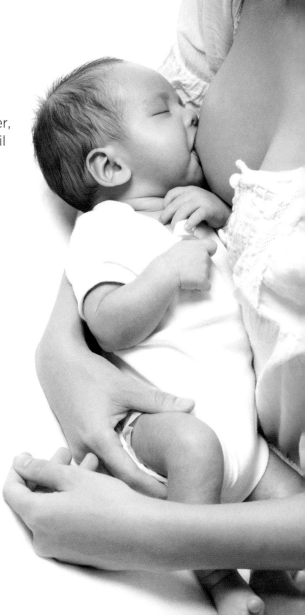

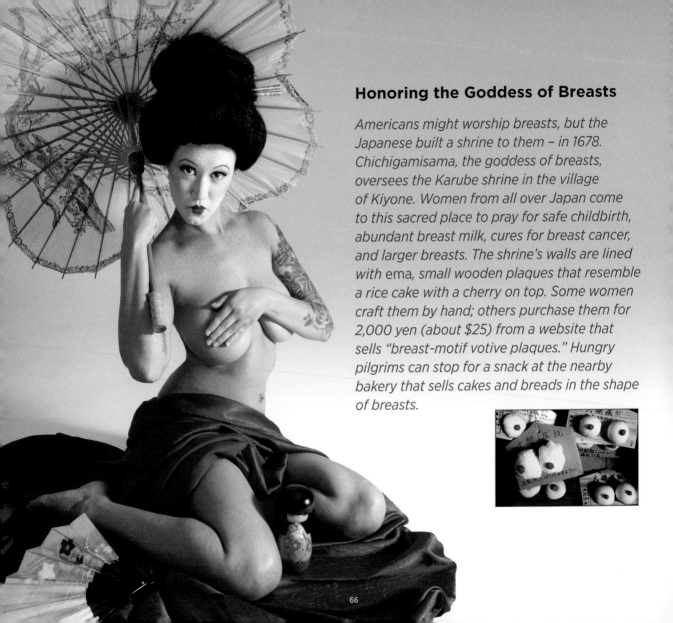

Honoring the Goddess of Breasts

Americans might worship breasts, but the Japanese built a shrine to them – in 1678. Chichigamisama, the goddess of breasts, oversees the Karube shrine in the village of Kiyone. Women from all over Japan come to this sacred place to pray for safe childbirth, abundant breast milk, cures for breast cancer, and larger breasts. The shrine's walls are lined with ema, small wooden plaques that resemble a rice cake with a cherry on top. Some women craft them by hand; others purchase them for 2,000 yen (about $25) from a website that sells "breast-motif votive plaques." Hungry pilgrims can stop for a snack at the nearby bakery that sells cakes and breads in the shape of breasts.

▶ Has Dr. Eisenberg ever operated on anyone with asthma, diabetes, or an overactive thyroid?

Yes, yes, yes. If your symptoms are under control, surgery is not a problem. As part of the presurgical workup, your breast health and general health are evaluated to make sure you can tolerate surgery, that you will heal well, and that surgery won't make your condition worse. If it's appropriate, your doctors will be contacted for medical clearance.

Diabetes can be monitored before and after surgery with a simple blood sugar test. A flare-up of asthma symptoms can be controlled with the patient's inhaler and a breathing treatment, if necessary. It is essential for a patient with an overactive thyroid (hyperthyroidism) to be under strict management because the condition can trigger heart irregularities, which may be difficult for the anesthesiologist to control during surgery.

▶ Can I have surgery if I have rheumatoid arthritis?

Although studies are ongoing, there are no reports in the current literature of a higher incidence of rheumatoid arthritis or other autoimmune diseases among women with breast implants. I tell women with a history of rheumatoid arthritis that implants could possibly aggravate their symptoms. I ask them to check with their rheumatologist to make sure he or she is supportive of their decision to have surgery. Most of these women choose to proceed with the operation; happily, no woman has reported that her symptoms got worse after surgery.

I'm in therapy. Does that matter?

Your mental health is as important as your physical health when you are considering cosmetic surgery. Just as I would ask your heart doctor for medical clearance, I would ask your therapist for clearance if you were currently in treatment or had received treatment recently.

I need to know that your therapist is supportive of your plans to have breast surgery at this time. It is necessary to have someone in your corner who knows the issues you are working on and can counsel you through your adjustment to your new body image.

◉◉ Titbit: "Primum non nocere" is a Latin phrase meaning, "First, do no harm." It is a fundamental principle of medicine and surgery that applies not just to elective cosmetic surgery but to any treatment.

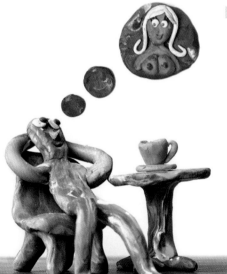

My boyfriend wants me to get breast implants. What do you think?

If you said this to me in consultation, I would ask if you wanted breast implants. If you said you were happy with how you look, I would tell you to go home. The surgery has to be for you, not to please someone else.

Only two women out of 5,000 have ever asked me this question. Although many men have the fantasy that women get implants to make them happy, they are wrong. Women primarily get implants to make themselves happy.

Sorry guys.

WHAT CAN YOU ACCOMPLISH?

▶ **My breasts are pointy and I don't like their shape.
Can you make them round?**

Implants will only make your breasts bigger and fuller; they won't change the shape of your breasts. You could compare breast augmentation to inflating a flat tire: When the tire on your car loses air, it loses some of its shape and it might appear to be flat. When you fill it up, it returns to its original shape.

It's essential to respect the anatomy of your breasts during surgery. If I tried to make your breasts wider, the implants might end up under your armpits. If I tried to lower the crease under your breasts, the implants might "bottom out," meaning you would have more breast fullness below your nipples than above them, and the nipples might look as if they were pointing toward the ceiling.

Not a good look.

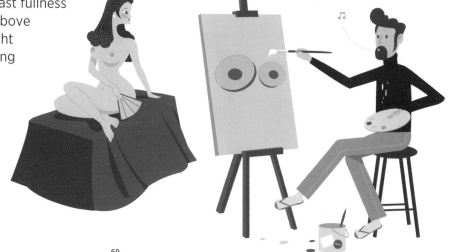

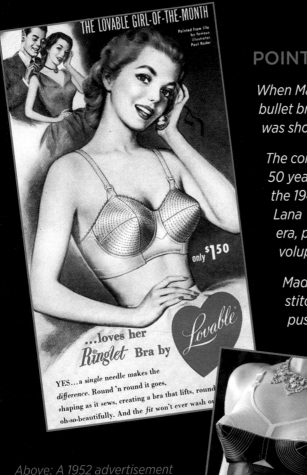

THE LOVABLE GIRL-OF-THE-MONTH

Painted from life
by famous
illustrator
Paul Rader

only $1.50

...loves her
Ringlet Bra by Lovable

YES...a *single* needle makes the
difference. Round 'n round it goes,
shaping as it sews, creating a bra that lifts, round
oh-so-beautifully. And the *fit* won't ever wash o...

*Above: A 1952 advertisement
for the Lovable Ringlet Bra.
Right: The Marlene Bullet Bra
from the vintage-inspired label
What Katie Did (www.whatkatiedid.us.com) "coaxes your
breasts into the perfect 1950's conical shape."*

POINTY BREASTS: A Fashion History

*When Madonna wore a Jean Paul Gaultier-designed
bullet bra during her 1990 Blond Ambition world tour, it
was shocking and erotic but not a new fashion concept.*

*The cone-shaped bullet bra had been popularized
50 years earlier by movie stars who came of age in
the 1940s, such as Marilyn Monroe, Jane Russell and
Lana Turner. They, along with the pinup girls of that
era, popularized the "Sweater Girl" look – pointy,
voluptuous breasts beneath a clingy sweater.*

*Made of nylon and satin and reinforced with circular
stitching around the cup, the bullet bra was the
push-up bra of its day. Women would iron their bras
to make sure the form was perfect and stuff the
cups for maximum projection.*

*The bullet bra, also known as the
torpedo bra, fell out of fashion in the
1960s when some women sought
a more natural look and others bought
the newest styles: underwire bras
and padded bras. These days, bullet
bras have made a comeback on
retro-lingerie websites.*

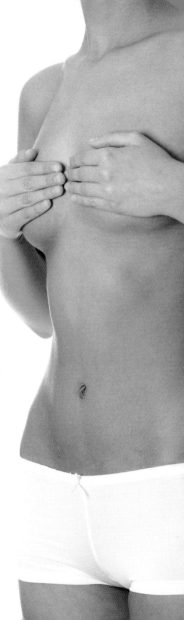

Can I go braless after I get implants?

Of course. There's no law against it. But if you imagine that your breasts will be perfectly symmetrical after surgery, you are dreaming. You will see improvement in and out of clothes, but subtle differences will still exist and possibly be visible when you are braless. If this is not a concern, then join the crowd: In August 2010, *Harper's Bazaar* reported on the new "peekaboob" fashion trend – perhaps started by French first lady Carla Bruni-Sarkozy, who had gone braless to a state dinner held in honor of Russian President Dmitry Medvedev five months earlier.

My breasts are different sizes. Can you even them out and make them exactly the same?

If there's a difference in the volume of your breasts, I can make them closer in size by enlarging them with implants of different sizes, augmenting the smaller breast, or reducing the bigger breast.

While I cannot transform your sisters into twins, I can make them look like sisters from the same family. I have operated on women whose breasts varied by as much as two cup sizes, and I was able to make a significant improvement.

⊙⊙ Titbit: While some women are bothered by a difference as small as a few tablespoons, others don't notice or don't care.

Will implants make my breasts look perky again?

If your breasts are mildly droopy, a saline or silicone gel implant placed behind the pectoral muscle might help create the illusion of perkiness. That's because as the implant fills out the top of the breast, it also fills out the bottom, making it look as if the nipple

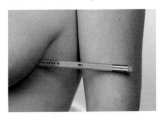

has moved higher. It hasn't. A silicone gel implant placed in front of the pectoral muscle might create the same illusion.

If your breasts are moderately to severely droopy and you get implants, it could look as if you have four breasts, with the breast implants up high and your natural breasts down low. A breast lift (mastopexy), with or without implants, would be a better choice; it would restore the breasts to a more youthful look by repositioning the nipples at a higher position and removing excess skin. To find out if you might be a candidate for a breast lift, turn to page 164 and take the "pencil test."

Do Your Boobs Hang Low?

Our camp counselors and Girl Scout leaders taught us the words to "Do Your Ears Hang Low?" But when they weren't around, we changed "ears" to "boobs" and sang it this way:

Do your boobs hang low? Do they wobble to and fro?
Can you tie them in a knot? Can you tie them in a bow?
Can you throw them over your shoulder like a Continental soldier?
Do your boobs hang low?

Exposing the Cover Up

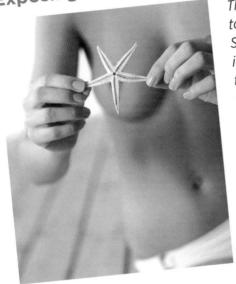

Thinking about going braless? How about topless? In many cities in the United States, women can be arrested and fined if they bare their breasts, which angers the folks at GoTopless.org. They assert that women have the same constitutional right as men to be bare-chested in public places. Each August, they organize an international Go Topless Day, where women protesters go bare and men wear bikini tops or bras to show their solidarity. Their motto:

"Free your breasts! Free your mind!"

On its website, GoTopless.org lists 14 cities that are "officially topless tested," including Austin, TX; Madison, WI; and Columbus, OH. The site advises: "Even if a top-free law is firmly in effect, the police can still arrest you under the pretense of disorderly conduct. Don't be intimidated! You can sue the city back for wrongful arrest if your only crime was to go topless."

▶ Will implants give me more cleavage?

Implants won't change the space between your breasts, but they will give you more breast volume, which will make it easier for you to enhance your cleavage with the right bra. If a surgeon tries to create or increase cleavage by loosening the inside borders – or going beyond the natural limits – of your breasts, you could end up with symmastia, also known as a uniboob. Again, not a good look.

Was He Singing About a Uniboob?

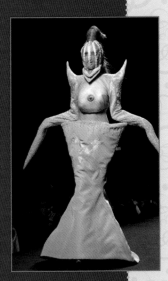

*"She's got one big breast in the middle of her chest
And an eye in the middle of her nose
So says I, if you look her in the eye
You're better off looking up her nose."*

– The Royal Nonesuch was a circus sideshow character in the Broadway musical Big River: The Adventures of Huckleberry Finn. *We wonder what inspired Roger Miller to write these lyrics. Did he and Gianni Molaro (see below) have the same bad dream?*

A Titter Went Round the Audience

Art couture designer Gianni Molaro shocked the crowd at Rome Fashion Week in January 2012 with his uniboob dress, officially titled "Fishlike Alien With a Literal Boob in the Center." Will this be Lady Gaga's next concert outfit?

Will I look natural? I don't want my breasts to look fake.

When breast implants are placed behind the pectoral muscle, the muscle blunts the part of the implant that peeks out of a tank top, bra or bathing suit, creating a more natural look. When saline breast implants are placed in front of the pectoral muscle, only skin and breast tissue camouflage the implants, and they might look unnatural, especially if a woman is very thin. Breasts might also look unnatural when the implants are too big for a woman's frame or are out of proportion with the rest of her body.

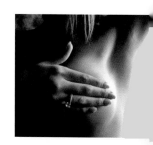

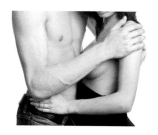

Will my breasts feel unnatural? Will people be able to tell by touching them?

Most implants are placed behind the chest muscle, so if someone touches your breast, he or she will feel your own breast tissue for the most part. It is common to be able to feel the implant on the side or underneath the breast, where there is little or no muscle coverage. The thinner you are, the easier it is to feel the implants, but it seems to be a nonissue for most women.

Will people notice that I got breast implants?

Patients tell me that their most observant friends and family members are often aware that something is different about them, but they can't pinpoint what it is. These curious people ask questions like, "You look great. Are you just back from vacation?" or "That's a cute outfit. Is it new?" Most women look natural and proportional after their breast augmentation surgery and can keep it a secret if they are so inclined. And if they are ever in the mood, they can choose to show off "the girls."

Clueless

Names have been changed to protect the enhanced:

Jennifer was in her early 20s and still living at home with her parents. She told her mom about her surgery, but she didn't want her dad to know. She was sure he would notice though; he was a surgeon, and she would be recuperating in the house for a week. She did not need to worry; her father was clueless.

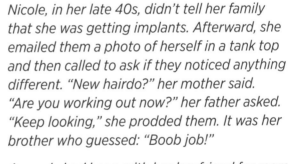

Nicole, in her late 40s, didn't tell her family that she was getting implants. Afterward, she emailed them a photo of herself in a tank top and then called to ask if they noticed anything different. "New hairdo?" her mother said. "Are you working out now?" her father asked. "Keep looking," she prodded them. It was her brother who guessed: "Boob job!"

Amanda had been with her boyfriend for more than a year. When he complimented her on her "perfect breasts," she simply said thank you. He didn't find out that she had implants until he looked through one of her old photo albums and saw a picture of her at the beach – before her surgery. He still thought her breasts were perfect!

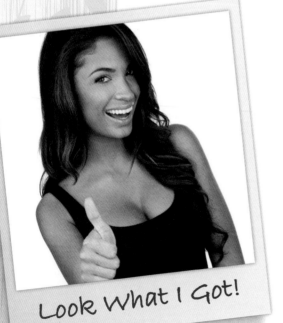

Look What I Got!

❱ Do implants cause stretch marks?

Usually, breast implants don't create new stretch marks. If you already have stretch marks, implants might make them less noticeable, temporarily redden them and make them more visible, or not change them at all.

❱ Will implants make my areolas larger?

Areolas normally remain the same size, but women who have had children sometimes think their areolas are larger after surgery. Here's why: During pregnancy, areolas often get darker and larger. Then, when the milk is gone and the breasts get smaller, it may look as if the areolas have shrunk. When implants restore the breasts' fullness, the areolas' post-pregnancy size again becomes apparent.

❱ Will my nipples stay erect all the time because the implants push them out?

There is a common misconception that nipples stay erect after breast augmentation surgery. It's an urban legend, no more real than the story about New York City's sewers being infested with deadly alligators.

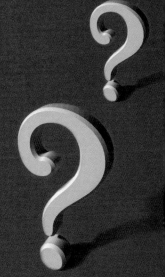

Implants don't affect the nipples. Sometimes, a woman doesn't realize that her nipples had the appearance of being erect before surgery. Now that her breasts are enlarged, it's more apparent to her, but the nipples have not actually changed. It's similar to the areola illusion. When women see their before-and-after photographs side by side, they are often surprised that their nipples haven't changed at all.

Will the weight of the implants make my breasts saggy?

In general, no. Most women opt for average-sized implants, which are not heavy enough to make breasts sag.

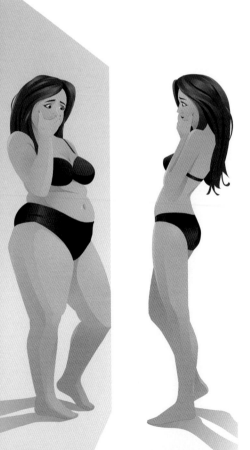

Will implants make me look fatter?

This is a common concern, but no woman has told me that she looked heavier after surgery. Women do tell me that their implants make them look more proportional, which means their figure might go from pear-shaped (or bottom-heavy) to hourglass-shaped.

My friend got breast implants (350 ccs) a few months ago and gained 10 pounds. Why?

Blame it on the cheesecake and the box of chocolates, not on her new breasts. If her implants are saline, her new pair weighs a total of about 1.5 pounds. If they are silicone gel, they are closer to 1.7 pounds. She can't use them as an excuse to stop her aerobic exercise either: She only needs to wait three weeks after surgery before starting up again.

To calculate how much your implants weigh, turn to page 81.

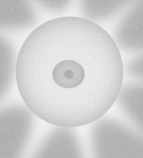

What will happen to my breasts if I get implants and later decide to take them out?

When implants are removed, breasts often return to their starting size (or close to it), much like a woman's stretched belly will generally go back to its original size after childbirth. The more elastic the skin, the greater the likelihood that it will shrink back to normal after it has been stretched.

Breast augmentation can make my life better, right?

No one comes right out and asks, but for some women it's an unspoken question. When I ask women what they are hoping to accomplish through breast surgery besides the physical change, they commonly say they want to "feel more womanly," "feel more feminine," and "have a little more self-confidence." If someone says, "I'm so unhappy and I need something to make me feel better," it raises concern. Breast implants don't change the issues in your life; they only change your appearance. They are not a shortcut to happiness.

"Looking at cleavage is like looking at the sun. You can't stare at it. It's too risky. You get a sense of it and then you look away."

- Jerry Seinfeld

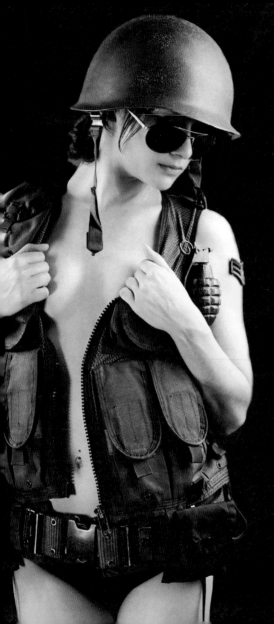

❱ Do you get a lot of exotic dancers?

My patients include bartenders, nurses, hairstylists, veterinarians, housecleaners, doctors, women who work on overhead power lines, teachers and students, flight attendants, exotic dancers (about 1%), nurses who have become exotic dancers, exotic dancers who have become nurses, ballroom dancers, stay-at-home moms, company executives, waitresses, fitness trainers, competitive bodybuilders, cheerleaders, policewomen who want to know how soon they can put their bulletproof vests back on, and women in all branches of the military who have emailed us from Iraq and Afghanistan to schedule appointments for when they are back in the United States. Of course, this is not a complete list.

❱ What will happen to my breasts when I turn 65?

They'll save $2 on a movie ticket and get a discounted cup of coffee at McDonald's. If as you age your breasts start to droop, the implants won't stay up high. They'll move south, too, right along with your breasts.

How Much Does Your Pair of Implants Weigh?

You Do the Math.

Step 1. Add the number of ccs in your right and left implants.

Step 2. If you have saline implants: Multiply the resulting number by .0325 (the weight of one ounce of saline). If you have silicone gel implants: Multiply the resulting number by .0375 (the weight of one ounce of silicone gel).

Step 3. Add 1.5 (the weight of the 2 implant shells in ounces).

Step 4. Divide by 16 (to adjust from ounces to pounds).

> **FOR EXAMPLE: If you have 400 cc saline implants:**
>
> **Step 1.** 400 + 400 = 800
>
> **Step 2.** 800 x .0325 = 26
>
> **Step 3.** 26 + 1.5 = 27.5
>
> **Step 4.** 27.5 ÷ 16 = **1.72 pounds**

HOW DO YOU GET THEM IN?

Where do you make the incision?

I make an incision in the inframammary fold (IMF), the crease below the breast where the breast and the chest meet. I then place the implant behind the breast tissue and the chest muscle. Although there are other approaches, I prefer this one because I don't have to touch nerves, blood vessels or breast tissue. The submuscular space (or pocket) is clearly visible, which allows me to easily stop any bleeding should it occur. I have used this approach for more than 5,000 breast augmentation patients, and I have found it to be safe and successful.

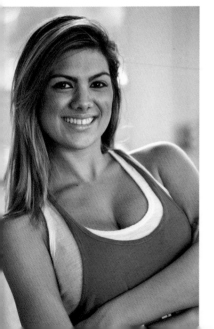

How big will the incision be?

For saline implants, the incision averages 1½ inches long; for silicone gel it's closer to 2 inches. Silicone gel implants are prefilled, so the surgeon needs to make a larger opening to insert them into the space. By contrast, saline implants come empty and can be folded up and inserted through a smaller incision.

How do you fill a saline implant?

Once the implant is in place but before the incision is closed, sterile saline solution is drawn out of an IV bag and into a filling syringe. The saline is inserted through a valve in the implant. The valve is self-sealing, which prevents the saline from leaking out.

Will the scar be noticeable?

Most women have some degree of crease under each breast, and I make the incision as close to the inframammary fold as possible in order to hide it. It's harder to hide an incision when a woman has little breast tissue and no crease, or when the distance from the nipple to the crease is very short. After the implants settle, the incision sometimes moves a little higher than the crease and can be visible when a woman is naked, but a bra or bathing suit will almost always hide it.

During a consultation, women see photos of the incision, and they can decide how they feel about it. It's rare that a woman decides not to get an augmentation because it means having a scar. Patients have told me that when they look at themselves in the mirror after surgery, they usually don't see the incision. They see their new proportional figure and they're pleased because that's what they wanted their surgery to accomplish.

⊙⊙ Titbit: If you have a scar from a previous surgery, it's usually an indicator of how you will heal. Most people heal well.

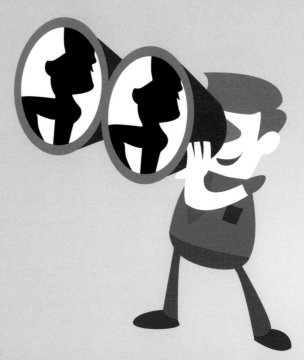

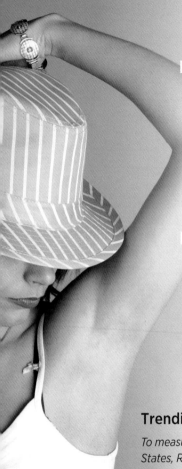

Can implants be put in through the armpit?

With the transaxillary approach, breast implants are put in place through an incision in the armpit. The implant passes close to blood vessels and nerves that run from the armpit to the chest. It's not common to injure these nerves, but doing so could cause hand and arm problems. If there is bleeding in the lower portion of the implant's space (the farthest point from the armpit), and if it's difficult to see and reach, the surgeon might have to make an incision under the breast to stop the bleeding.

Can implants be put in through the nipple?

In the periareolar approach, an incision is made along the outline of the areola. The breast implant passes near nerves leading to the nipple, which could lessen sensitivity and cause interference with breastfeeding later on. The implant is also passed near milk ducts. If bacteria normally found in the milk ducts come in contact with an implant, there could be an increased chance of infection. Often, the scar blends in with the areola; if a patient doesn't heal well, it will be visible.

Trending Now in Salt Lake City: Breast Implants

To measure women's interest in breast implants across the United States, RealSelf.com analyzed millions of searches on its website by region. (They assumed that women were doing the searching.) Compared with the national average, interest in breast implants was highest in the cities listed at right. The women of Columbia, SC, showed the least interest in breast implants, followed by those in Baltimore, Boston and Washington, DC.

1.	Salt Lake City, UT	+74%
2.	Fresno, CA	+63%
3.	Honolulu, HI	+54%
4.	Oklahoma City, OK	+50%
5.	Mobile, AL	+34%

What is scarless breast augmentation?

It is another name for transumbilical breast augmentation (TUBA). The incision is made inside the belly button, and implants are tunneled up to the breasts. Only saline implants can be placed with this approach; silicone gel implants, which are prefilled before insertion, can't fit through the tunnels.

Can you take the extra fat from my butt and put it in my breasts?

As early as the 1920s, doctors attempted to enlarge breasts with fatty tissue taken from the stomach and buttock areas. Within a year the body would reabsorb most of the fat, and the breasts could get lumpy and uneven. The approach was abandoned in 1940. When liposuction was developed in the 1970s, some doctors took the liposuctioned fat and injected it into the breasts. More success was achieved with this method, but it still had some limitations.

The latest approach is to mix a woman's fat with her stem cells before injecting it into the breast. Although the results may be longer-lasting, the amount of enlargement is somewhat modest. The technique is also useful for repairing small areas with defects after breast cancer surgery.

I HAD NO IDEA . . .

When staff members Pat Smith, Eileen Ricciutti, Nan McCarthy, Sharon Sisle and Gerry Gorgol joined my team, working in a cosmetic breast surgery practice was new for all of them. We asked them what surprised them and what they have learned on the job. Here's what they said:

Pat, *Accounting Coordinator*

Before I started to work here, I had seen very few breasts. I didn't have any sisters. We didn't get undressed in front of each other in gym class; we didn't talk about our breasts or look at each other's. I think this is the case for most women.

I never knew that girls had concerns – that one breast might be smaller than the other, or that one might point down and the other up. I didn't know why women would get breast implants; I thought it might be a fad. Now I understand.

Nan, *Patient Coordinator*

When I started my job, I had the misconception that only strippers and celebrities got breast implants. I wondered: How busy could the office be? How many women would get this done? You'd be surprised. I take it all back. I had no idea that regular women had cosmetic breast surgery. I was shocked by what I saw when women came in for an appointment and took off their bras. Many women didn't have much of anything there.

I love my job. When women call for appointments, they tell me how they feel about their breasts. They have similar feelings, but each woman expresses it in a different way. They try to give me a good reason why they want breast surgery. I get it. We all do.

Gerry, *Patient Facilitator*

I didn't know anyone who had cosmetic breast surgery, and I was actually shocked when I saw that some women have a small A cup on one side and a B or C cup on the other. I didn't know that existed.

I really enjoy being in the room when Dr. Eisenberg meets with and examines patients. Everyone has a different story and a different outlook; their reactions to what he tells them are so interesting. It's been a great learning experience.

Sharon, *Facility Coordinator and Patient Facilitator*

I thought I knew who got breast implants, so I was really surprised when I met the women who were coming in for surgery. These women are like me; they could be my daughters or my friends. And when I am in the exam room and see what women live with, I wonder why insurance doesn't pay for cosmetic breast surgery.

In the office, I'm responsible for the before-and-after photo books and for printing out everyone's pictures. When I see the photos, I see what a difference surgery can make. The results are amazing. It is truly life-changing.

Eileen, *Financial and Surgical Coordinator*

I thought that only dancers and women who wanted new boyfriends or husbands got breast implants, but I quickly discovered that this is not the case at all. Women tell me that their partners love them exactly how they are, and they are having surgery to make themselves look and feel better. That's their motivation. I see how happy women are after surgery and how great they look in their clothes. It gives them a big boost.

I never had such intimate conversations with people until I came to work here. When women discover they can talk to us about their breasts, they lighten up and loosen up. It's like talking to a girlfriend. Before they hang up, they often say, "I feel as if I've known you forever; I can't wait to meet you."

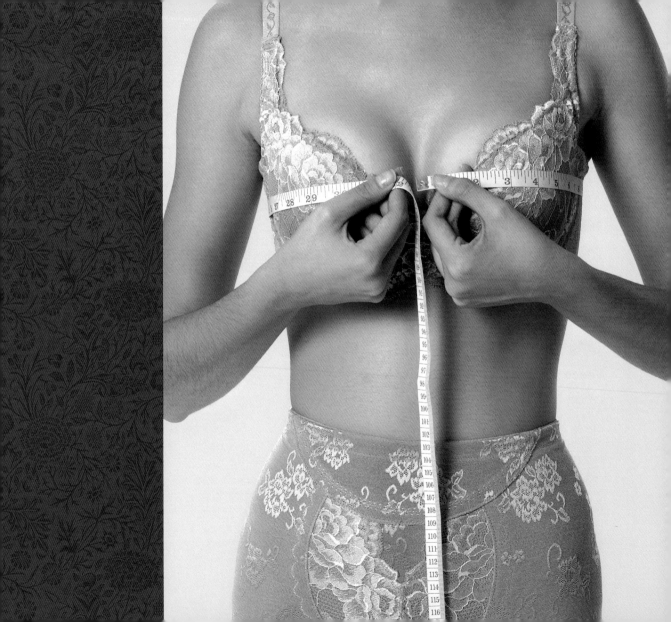

Chapter 4

Size Matters

*"Do you want to be proportional,
turn heads or stop traffic?"*

That's what one of my colleagues asks a prospective breast augmentation
patient to see what she has in mind. I've tried it. Most women tell me they
want to be proportional; some comment that they wouldn't mind turning heads
now and then. Not many want to stop traffic. Ironically, some of my patients are
policewomen who literally stop traffic – but they would rather
not do it with their breasts.

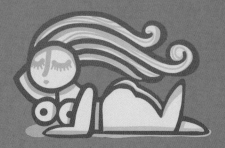

❱ Can you make me proportional?

Yes, but you need to tell me what proportional means to you. Some women say, "I've got the bottom half of the hourglass, and I need something up top to balance it out." Others have small breasts and narrow hips and just want "anything up top so I feel more like a woman."

Throughout history and across cultures, the beauty ideal has changed. Italian Renaissance painter Raphael depicted women with small breasts and large, curvaceous hips, the ideal proportions in the early 1500s. Victoria's Secret models – the contemporary icons of beauty – have large breasts, tiny waists and tight hips.

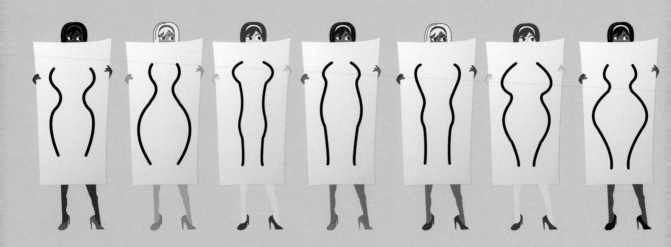

Are You a Pear or an Apple?

The most sought-after shape in modern times is the hourglass figure, described as equal hip and bust measurements and a narrow waist. Marilyn Monroe, who measured 35-22-35, was its personification. In a 2005 study of American body types, researchers found that the ideal is rarely achieved:

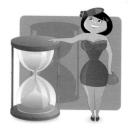

- *Only 8% of women had hourglass figures.*

- *14% were apple-shaped (top heavy).*

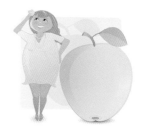

- *20% were pear-shaped (bottom heavy).*

- *46% were banana-shaped, minus the curve (straight).*

That leaves 12 percent of women unaccounted for. Perhaps they fall somewhere else on the list of the body shapes identified by Trinny & Susannah, British fashion advisors and hosts of the BBC's What Not to Wear *TV show. Along with the shapes noted above, their list includes vase, cello, ice cream cone, lollipop, column, bowling pin, bell, goblet and brick shapes.*

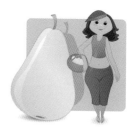

❯ Can you make me a full C cup?

Most women think that being proportional means wearing a C cup bra. By and large (pun intended), they tell me that they want to be "a full C cup – *not* a D!" To them, D is the size of their grandmother's bra, but a C cup could mean one thing if it's made by Victoria's Secret and another if it's made by Vanity Fair. You might wear a B cup in a

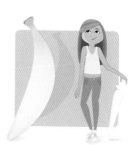

(continued)

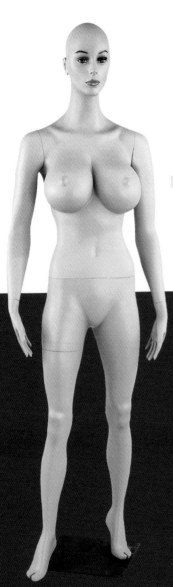

full-coverage bra and a C cup in a demi bra, even if the same company makes both styles. Because there is no standard cup-sizing system, I prefer to call it a C look. To achieve a C look, a 5-foot woman with a small frame might need a B cup while a 5-foot-8-inch woman with a large frame might need a D cup.

What implant size is equal to a C cup?

Breast implants are measured in cubic centimeters (ccs), not cup size. On a woman who is completely flat-chested and has a medium-sized frame, a 450 cc implant would be equivalent to the average C-cup bra.

They Look So Fake!

The large majority of women who come to me for breast augmentation want to look proportional, but mannequin makers have apparently not gotten the memo. While the classic female mannequin has a small B cup, manufacturers are now selling "sexy/busty mannequins" and "voluptuous female mannequins" with 40DDs and Barbie doll-sized waists. Apparently, sales are through the roof. You can find these well-endowed plastic women in boutique windows from SoHo to South Beach.

AFTER   BEFORE

▶ My girlfriend got 375 cc implants. Can I get that size, too?

Yes, but keep in mind that you need to compare apples to apples, so to speak. If you're starting with a full B cup and your girlfriend started with a mid-A, you won't end up the same size when you both get 375 cc implants. You'll be about one cup-size bigger – the extra cup you started with.

▶ I saw photos online of a woman with 325 cc implants, and she looked great. Can you order those for me?

There are several problems with picking your implant size from online photos. The woman you are admiring might have started out with breasts that were larger or smaller than yours, and she might be a different height and weight.

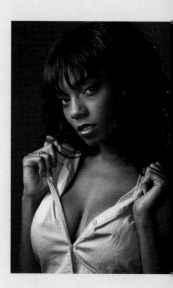

If the pictures are not labeled, you don't know how far along she is in the healing process. If you are looking at photos taken three months after surgery, consider this: The implants are not yet settled into their final position. They are pressed up high, like your breasts would be in a push-up bra. At nine months when they settle, they will have the illusion of looking smaller. You might be disappointed if you choose your implant size from pictures taken three months after surgery.

▶ I want to be a D. Can you fit that much in?

Maybe. Larger implants are greater in both volume and width. There is a limit to how large an implant can fit behind the chest muscle, and it's dependent on the width of each breast – the distance from the side of the breastbone to the outside of the breast.

(continued)

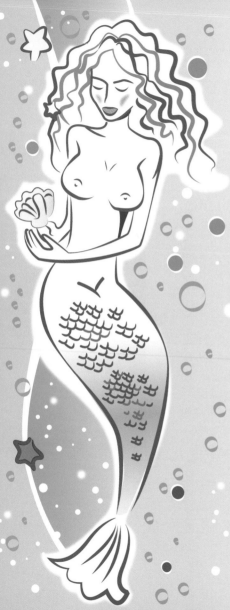

Over time, the muscle relaxes, the skin stretches, and the implants settle down. Then there may be room to insert larger implants. After at least nine months, women can opt to have a second operation to go bigger.

My oldest patient was 63. She's also the patient who requested the largest implants – equivalent to a double D. She understood that her frame couldn't accommodate all that she wanted during the first surgery, so she waited about a year and then had a second operation.

Mermaid Makeover

After two years of debate about the ideal size and shape of mermaid breasts, the town council of Ustka, Poland, voted to augment the breast size of the mermaid on its coat of arms. The goal was to boost tourism. The original 1922 symbol was small-busted and nipple-less; the 2006 makeover gave her fuller breasts, nipples, and flowing curls (think Disney's Ariel).

BEFORE

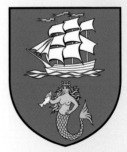

AFTER

**I'm getting 400 cc implants, but my girlfriend says her 400 cc implants are too big and I should get 375 ccs instead.
What do you think?**

I think you should cover your ears and disregard her well-meaning advice. The difference between a 375 cc and a 400 cc implant is less than 2 tablespoons – the amount of oil you would add to your boxed pancake mix. Plus, your friend's starting size might have been different from yours.

After you've chosen the size that seems right to you, consider that you are the expert on what you like. Don't let your girlfriends and Internet forums confuse you.

Don't let your male friends confuse you, either. They might suggest that you get larger implants. A plastic surgeon and a psychologist surveyed more than 34,000 people to find out what makes the female figure attractive and to determine if men and women judge the female body differently. Their results, published in *Aesthetic Plastic Surgery*, showed that women prefer slightly wider hips, a narrower waist, and longer legs than men do. There was a clear difference in regard to the ideal bust size: 40 percent of men but only 25 percent of women preferred a large bust.

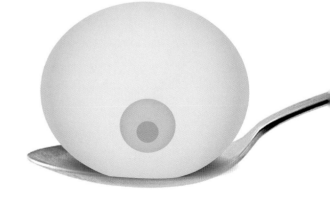

Should I put a bag of birdseed in my bra to see how I'll look with bigger breasts? What about breast sizers?

You could slip zip-lock bags filled with rice or birdseed into your bra to get an idea of how you'll look with bigger breasts. You could also try breast implant sizers, which are less scratchy and better conform to your breasts. Sizer kits come with a special bra and silicone gel or saline implants in a range of cubic centimeters; you can try implants of various sizes under different clothes to see what size you prefer. The saline implants come empty; you'll have to fill them using the accompanying syringe. Luckily, there's a plug to stop leaks.

If you stuff your bra with Minute Rice and look in the mirror, what you see is not what you'll get when that same volume is placed behind the pectoral muscle. Your breasts will look smaller because the muscle flattens the implant. When you say, "I want to have the same look that I have in this bra, with this sizer or this bag of birdseed," your surgeon has to draw on his or her experience and judgment to determine how many cubic centimeters are needed to accomplish your goal.

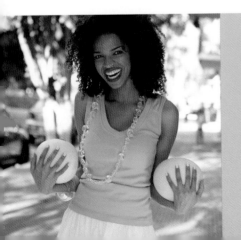

Check Out Those Melons!

When the folks at IntimateGuide.com heard about a man who walked into a lingerie shop and said, "I need a bra for my girlfriend; she's about the size of a grapefruit," they decided to find out how fruit size actually correlates to bra size.

Here's what they found:

Lemons and kiwis = A cup. Apples = B cup. Oranges = C cup. Grapefruits = D cup. Melons = DDD cup.

Do Vietnamese Bikers Measure Up?

In 2008, in a peculiar attempt to make their roads safer, the Vietnamese government proposed banning anyone who was too short, too thin, too sickly, or too small-chested (under 28 inches) from riding a motorbike on public roads. Before the traffic police had to pull over drivers to measure their chests, the proposal was defeated. Perhaps it was a scheme to sell more padded bras.

⊙⊙Titbit:
Ten years ago, my patients chose 350 cc saline implants on average. Now, the average is 425 ccs.

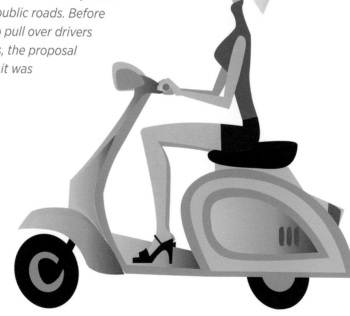

▶ How do I know what size implants to get?

During consultations, I show prospective patients before-and-after photographs of women who started out similar to them in height, weight, frame size and breast volume. Every photo notes the size of the implants that were used. Women vote on the breast sizes they see and tell me, "too big," too small" or "just right." It's like looking through a magic mirror into the future. Each women is consistent with her votes on the number of cubic centimeters (ccs) she likes, so I know what size implant will give her the look she wants on her body.

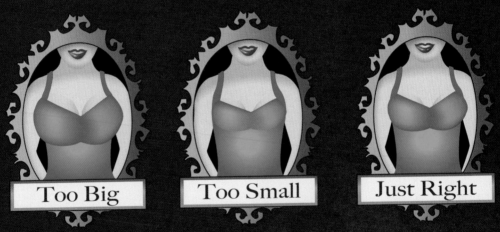

Too Big   Too Small   Just Right

When we are finished the process, women almost always ask, "What cup size will I be? If my answer is "D," they often say, "I don't want to be a D. Show me something smaller." This is where they get into trouble. The letter doesn't matter. They chose a look, and it looked right to them. Women should trust themselves; I trust that they know what they like.

Do you do 3-D breast imaging?

No. I prefer using my before-and-after photos, but here's how imaging works: After three-dimensional photos of your breasts are taken, a computer program calculates their volume and dimensions and then simulates how you'll look with breast implants of various sizes. Women shouldn't expect to look exactly as they do in their 3-D image. That's because, with the current technology, the simulation doesn't reflect whether the implant is in front of or behind the muscle, which makes a significant difference in the final result. Again, it's up to the surgeon to use his or her experience to convert the 3-D imaging data into cubic centimeters.

Will bigger breasts help me get a job?

They will probably help you land a job at a "breastaurant," the term for a restaurant that features scantily clad women. Hooters got the party started in 1983; since then Twin Peaks, Tilted Kilt and Mugs N Jugs have all tried to get in on the action.

Bigger breasts might also give you some opportunities in Italy: In 2008, Prime Minister Silvio Berlusconi selected Mara Carfagna, a topless model and actress, to be his Minister for Equal Opportunities.

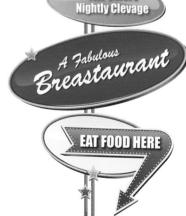

Debrahlee Lorenzana, a business banking officer at Citibank, had less luck with her double D breast implants. She was fired in 2010 for allegedly flaunting her curves. Lorenzana says she dressed professionally – no cleavage showing – but the company claimed that male co-workers were distracted by her too-sexy outfits. They asked her to tone it down and to avoid clingy sweaters and fitted suits. She complained about sexual harassment. Not long after, she was fired because she "wasn't fit for the culture of Citibank."

Covering Your A$$ets

1,000,000,000,000

Holly Madison, former star of The Girls Next Door and former girlfriend of Playboy magazine founder Hugh Hefner, took out a $1 million insurance policy on her breasts with Lloyd's of London when she got the starring role in Peepshow, a topless Las Vegas revue. "They're my primary moneymakers right now. If anything happened to my boobs, I'd be out for a few months and I'd probably be out a million dollars," she explained.

UNITED STATES OF AMERICA
One Trillion Dollars

Insuring one's assets is not a new idea.
Ben Turpin, a cross-eyed star of the silent movie era, took out a policy that would pay him if his eyes ever became uncrossed. That was in 1928. Since then, policies have been written on the rear end of a Brazilian model, the taste buds of a food critic, and the mustache of a cricket player. Also insured are Bruce Springsteen's voice, Mariah Carey's legs, and all of David Beckham. Dolly (Parton) insured her breasts years before Holly did.

⊙⊙ Titbit:
They call it a Bo-Tax: Looking for a solution to its budget deficit, the state of New Jersey slapped a 6 percent tax on elective cosmetic surgical procedures in 2004. The plan cost more than it brought in, and in 2012 a bill was passed to phase out the tax. Nevertheless, Connecticut passed a Bo-Tax in 2011, and proposals have been introduced in other state legislatures.

❱ Will I get better tips if I have bigger breasts?

Wouldn't you know that some guy researched this topic in depth? Cornell University Professor Michael Lynn surveyed 374 waitresses and discovered that those with larger breasts received bigger tips – as did women with blond hair and slender bodies. He also found that men gave women in their 30s the best tips, possibly "because they thought they had a better chance of picking up the older waitresses."

Bigger Breasts, Bigger Paycheck?

It depends on your job. For cocktail waitress Carol Ann Doda, it paved the way to riches. One of the country's first topless dancers, Doda bared all as she danced atop a white baby grand piano at the Condor Club in San Francisco in 1964. She was hugely popular – even before a gynecologist injected silicone into her size-34 breasts. Afterward, her 44Ds were known as "the new Twin Peaks of San Francisco," and a cartoon of her was painted on the strip club's marquee. Doda got a bigger paycheck and a bigger workload: She danced 12 shows a night.

LOOKING NATURAL

For most women, the goal of breast augmentation surgery is to look natural. Here's what they have told me about how they feel and what they would like surgery to accomplish:

- "It's pretty bad when your 13-year-old sister can already wear your bra."

- "I feel gypped. I've been a size 34A since eighth grade."

- "I never go on vacation unless it is to the mountains in the winter because I'm too embarrassed to wear a bathing suit."

- "I wear a size 32A and don't even fill that up. All of my bras and bathing suit tops are padded. Many times I've unknowingly walked around with one side of my bra pushed in, wondering why people were staring at me."

- "I want to like what I see in the mirror."

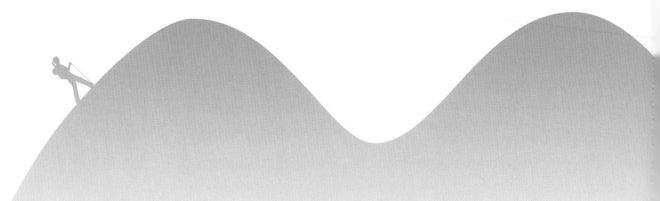

- *"I want to be made proportional."*

- *"I have dreamed of the day I could go to the beach with confidence or make love to my boyfriend with the lights on, while I was naked."*

- *"I don't want to be huge for some man; I want to be normal for myself."*

- *"I don't want to look like I'm falling over when I come into a room."*

- *"I don't want to look like an exotic dancer."*

- *"I'm paying a lot of money, so I want to make sure I go big enough."*

- *"I don't want people to notice."*

- *"I don't want to be perfect; I want to be me again."*

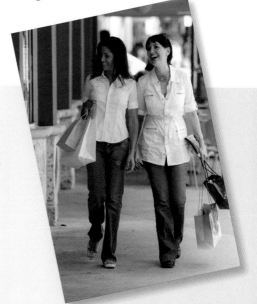

All in the Family

I have been performing cosmetic breast surgery long enough to have operated on dozens of mothers and their daughters. Sometimes, a mother has surgery first, and she is empathetic and supportive when her daughter comes of age and expresses interest. Other times, after a daughter has surgery, her mother sees how great she looks and decides to finally go for it herself.

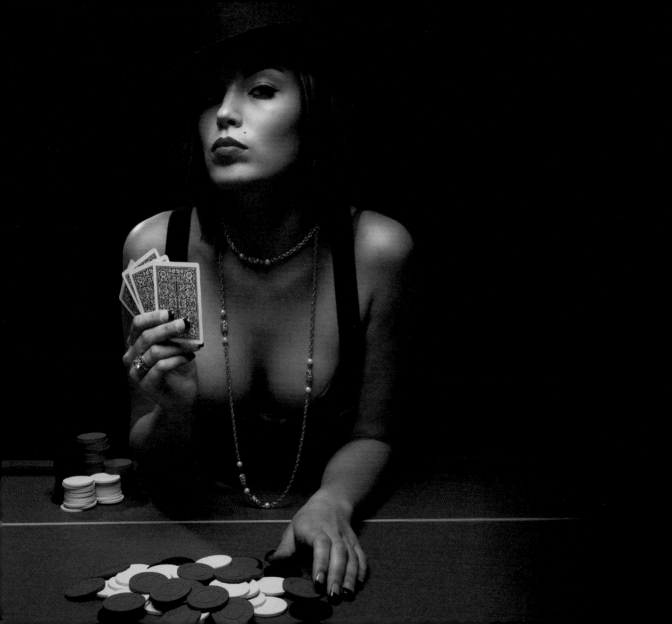

Chapter 5

Tits & Ask

Time to get down to business – to meet the doctor,
get your questions answered, find out if the surgical results could meet
your expectations, and talk price.

Consider this our T&A Q&A.

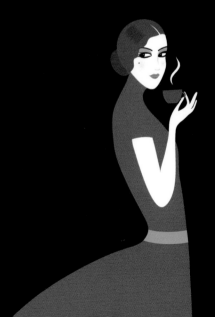

THE CONSULTATION

❯ Do I have to come in for a consultation before I have surgery?

Yes. Even though you may have read all about breast augmentation online and talked to your friends about their experience with surgery, you still need to have an in-person consultation to find out if there's a match between your goals and expectations and what the surgeon can accomplish.

❯ How soon after a consultation can I have surgery? Can I do it the same day?

Almost. In my practice, the shortest time ever between consultation and surgery was 17 hours. Before she came in for her consultation, this out-of-town patient:

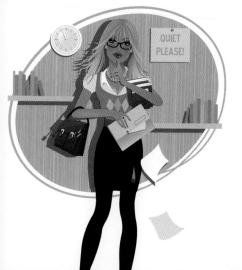

- sent us her medical information and a mammography report (not all patients need a mammogram),

- selected a surgery date and paid in full,

- completed a phone interview with a nurse from the hospital,

- had the required laboratory tests, and

- spoke with the anesthesiologist.

At her consultation, I determined that she was a suitable candidate for surgery, and she decided that I could meet her expectations. If we hadn't made a match, the surgery would have been canceled.

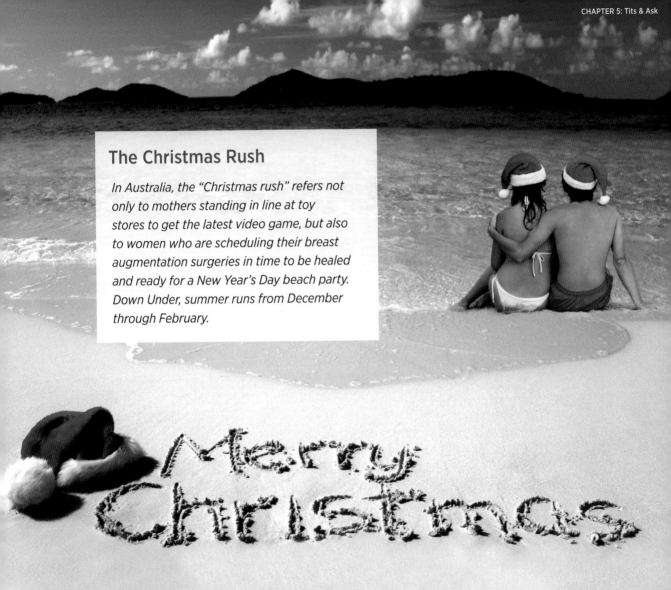

The Christmas Rush

In Australia, the "Christmas rush" refers not only to mothers standing in line at toy stores to get the latest video game, but also to women who are scheduling their breast augmentation surgeries in time to be healed and ready for a New Year's Day beach party. Down Under, summer runs from December through February.

❱ How much is a consultation?

Some surgeons offer a free consultation and others charge a fee, which may range from $75 to $250. Oftentimes, if you go ahead with the procedure, the consultation fee will be deducted from the cost of the surgery.

I offer free consultations because I know that prospective patients like to shop around. I want women to come in, meet us, and see what we have to offer. We pride ourselves on customer service, and accurate and honest information is the best service we can provide. It's like a first date: We try to make a good impression, so you will ask us out again.

❱ How long is a consultation?

Consultations commonly range from 30 to 60 minutes. You'll have a chance to talk about your expectations and find out what the surgery can accomplish. The doctor will take your medical history, discuss your specific health considerations, examine and measure your breasts, and talk to you about the surgical approach that's best for you. Together, you'll consider implant sizes and styles. Finally, you'll get the details of the procedure, review the risks of surgery, and learn what you can expect during the recovery period. Coincidentally, my patients generally spend the same amount of time in the consultation room as they do in the operating room – 43 minutes on average.

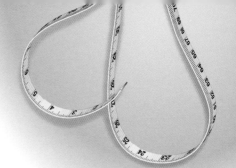

Taking Full Measure

*Although you might be focused on the size and shape of
your breasts, your surgeon has much more to evaluate, such as:*

- *Skin elasticity*
- *Breast diameter (the distance from 3 o'clock to 9 o'clock on each breast)*
- *The distance from the nipple to the crease under the breast (the amount of droop)*
- *Body type (small, medium or large-boned)*
- *Height and weight*

❱ Who's going to do my surgery?

That's a fair question. In my practice, I'm your doctor from start to finish. In a teaching
hospital, it's likely that a resident or fellow might be doing a portion of your surgery
under the supervision of the attending surgeon.

Sometimes, cosmetic surgery companies and large surgical centers subcontract with
surgeons to perform the procedures for which they advertise. In those cases, the doctor
who does your consultation might not be the doctor who performs your surgery.

❱ What does board-certified mean?

Board certification means recognition by one's peers of competency in a particular
medical specialty. It's not mandatory: Physicians can legally practice medicine by being
licensed by the state in which they practice. State laws differ, but licensure generally

(continued)

requires graduation from an accredited medical school in the United States or Canada, at least one year of postgraduate hospital training in an accredited residency program, and a passing score on a national board examination.

After physicians have completed an approved specialty training program and practiced that specialty for several years, they can pursue board certification. To demonstrate expertise, they must pass a rigorous written and oral examination administered by a medical specialty board. Some hospitals make board certification a prerequisite for physicians who want to join their staff.

Can my girlfriend and I come in together for a consultation?

Yes. Girls often go to the bathroom in pairs, and it's fairly common for girlfriends, sisters and cousins – and occasionally mothers and daughters – to schedule their consultations at the same time. Some women also schedule their surgeries on the same day, so they can recuperate together. Others choose to have surgery a few weeks apart, so they can take care of each other during the recovery period. Occasionally, a woman might be nervous and want her friend to go first, so she can see how it goes.

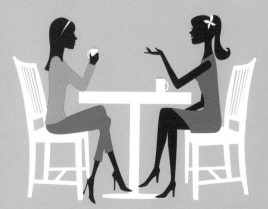

Although we don't assume that women want to be examined and measured together, they often do. They can also sit together while each reviews before-and-after photos and considers implant size. Surgical goals are an individual preference; even if both women want to be a full C, the implants needed to accomplish that look will vary depending on their body frame, height and weight.

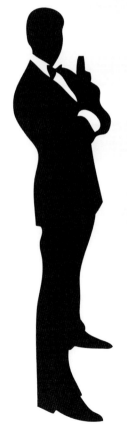

▶ What should I tell my children?

How about, "Mommy made a wish to the boob fairy"? After all, there is a tooth fairy. And who knows what would happen if you left your bra beneath your pillow?

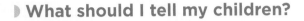

Some mothers are more forthright than others, depending on their willingness to reveal personal information and the age of their children. One mother explained it to her child this way: "When I had a baby, my breasts disappeared, and I'm going to the doctor's office to get them back."

Most women think their children will notice the change. Some do and some don't. In a post on BreastImplants4You.com, one mother said she told her 8-year-old daughter that she was having surgery to remove some moles. "The day after my surgery she came up to me while I was resting and looked at my chest. She said, 'Mom, look how lucky you are! When they removed your moles, your boobies got bigger.' "

▶ What size implants did my friend get?

The HIPAA Privacy Rule prevents me from mentioning the names of my patients. So when a woman asks me a question like this or tells me that her sister says hello, I say, "You can mention her name, but I can't reveal that I even know her." I would make a superb secret agent.

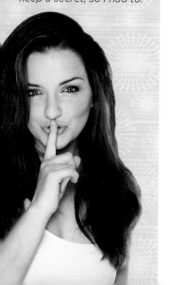

Does the doctor's wife have implants?

I don't tell my wife the names of the women who get implants – and some of them are women she knows – and I wouldn't tell my patients if my wife had implants. When I refuse to answer, women often ask the question another way: "If your wife or daughter wanted implants, would you be supportive?" The answer is yes.

Note from the doctor's wife: "I'm happy with my natural breast size, but if I wanted implants, I would choose Dr. Eisenberg!"

I'm not telling my husband about my augmentation. How do I keep him from knowing?

To keep him in the dark, you'll need to find some reasons to keep your lights off and your clothes on. You won't be the only woman doing this: In a 2010 survey conducted by MyCelebrityFashion.co.uk, 61 percent of the 1,563 women polled preferred sex with the lights off, and 48 percent preferred to wear at least one garment during sex. For most of these women, it was their bra.

I've Got a Secret, Too

Lauren (not her real name) got implants when she was married to her first husband. When she remarried, she kept it a secret from her second husband, which created a challenge when she decided to get bigger implants. Husband No. 2 thought it was her first surgery and asked to come to the consultation with her. When Lauren called to schedule her appointment, she asked us to pretend that we had never met her.

"I was going to have cosmetic surgery until I noticed that the doctor's office was full of portraits by Picasso."

– Rita Rudner

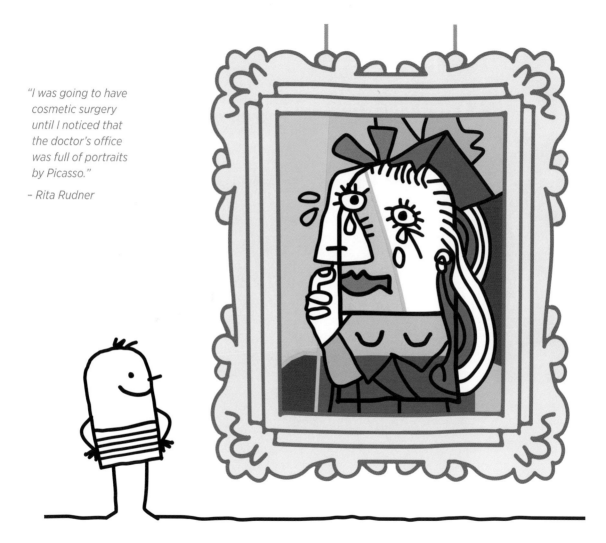

THE COST

▶ How much does breast augmentation cost?

Around the country, the total cost of breast augmentation falls between $4,000 and $10,000. Doctors commonly charge about $1,000 more for silicone gel implants than for saline implants. That's because silicone gel implants are more expensive to produce, and manufacturers pass that cost along to doctors, who pass it along to patients.

▶ Is it more expensive to get bigger implants?

It's rare for surgeons to charge more for a breast augmentation with larger-sized implants. Manufacturers don't charge by the cubic centimeter either: They charge one set price for all off-the-shelf saline breast implants, whether they are 200 ccs or 600 ccs, and another set price (about $1,000 higher) for silicone gel implants.

"B is for Breasts, Of which ladies have two;
Once prized for the function, Now for the view."

– Robert Paul Smith, American author

❱ Does the price include anesthesia?

It's important to ask this question because the quoted price sometimes includes only the surgeon's fee. Be sure to ask what you're getting for your money. At my office, the price is all-inclusive. It includes the surgical fee, implants (yes, two of them), anesthesia, laboratory tests, use of the operating room, all follow-up visits, and a 10-year warranty for deflation.

❱ Are breast implants cheaper in Costa Rica?

Maybe. If you're looking for an all-inclusive cosmetic surgery package that includes beach volleyball and an open bar, you can travel abroad, get breast implants, and spend a week recuperating at a tropical resort. The actual procedure will probably cost less, but you'll have to factor in the costs of a round-trip flight and your hotel stay.

In recent years, travel companies have sprung up to facilitate medical tourism. Agents book your hotel and flights, guide you through the paperwork, schedule your consultation and procedure, and arrange for someone to greet you at the airport. But whether you have surgery in Maine or Mexico, it's essential to do your due diligence: Inquire about the surgeon's credentials, the facility's accreditation, and the plans for your follow-up care.

Medical tourism has a long history. For thousands of years, people have traveled to Japan for its mineral springs and to India for its ancient healing traditions. Travel for cosmetic surgery

⊙⊙ Titbit: Don't think that medical tourism is a one-way street. Consumers from Great Britain and Europe, encouraged by the attractive exchange rate for their pounds and euros, are booking trips to the U.S. solely for cosmetic surgery.

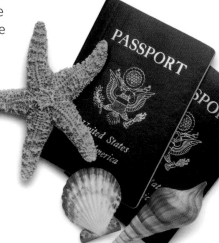

(continued)

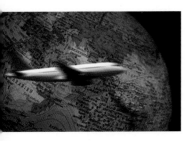

and dentistry is a more recent phenomenon, spurred on by rising health care costs. After Thailand's economic troubles in the late 1990s, the government marketed the country as a top destination for plastic surgery. Now, countries ranging from Brazil and Costa Rica to Turkey and the United Arab Emirates have gotten in on the action. It's estimated that between 100,000 and 200,000 Americans travel across international borders each year for medical care.

▶ Will my health insurance cover the surgery?

Cosmetic surgery procedures, such as breast augmentation and breast lift, are considered elective surgeries and are not covered by health insurance. Breast reduction surgery may be covered if your insurance company agrees that it is medically necessary. Health insurance companies pay for breast reconstruction surgery after a mastectomy.

▶ How does financing work?

Surgical loan companies offer a variety of financing plans that allow you to make monthly payments, sometimes with no money down. The interest rate is based on your credit history. You can call a company and find out if you are approved in just 10 minutes – even before you come in for a consultation.

▶ Can I send in $1,000 at a time until I have paid in full?

Yes, as long as the fee is fully paid before surgery. Some women do send weekly or monthly payments to us instead of making a one-time payment. If you can purchase your furniture on layaway, why not your new breasts?

Can my ex-husband mail you a check?

Although many women pay for their own breast implants, we have also encountered plenty of "angel investors" who provide capital for a breast perk-up: parents, stepparents, husbands, fiancés, boyfriends, girlfriends who are friends, girlfriends who are partners, siblings, bosses, co-workers, ex-spouses, and clients of dancers and strippers. Occasionally a woman brings her client, rather than her husband, to her appointments.

Why do I have to pay for surgery in advance?

Because unlike cars, houses, or 52-inch flat-screen televisions, breast implants can't be repossessed if you don't pay your bill.

Wanted: The Owner of These Breasts

Dr. Michael Koenig, a plastic surgeon in Cologne, Germany, was fed up with patients who registered under fake names and ran away right after their surgeries without paying. One woman stepped out "to get some fresh air" and never came back. Dr. Koenig made posters of these patients' augmented breasts and gave them to the police in the hopes that the fugitives could be found. He now demands payment in advance.

Will you take my diamond ring for payment?

"Can I give you the title to my car?" "Can I build a custom entertainment center for you?" Thanks for asking, but we don't barter or accept payments other than cash, checks, money orders,

(continued)

direct wire deposits, credit cards, and payments from health care financing companies. How women get their money together is up to them. We have been paid in stacks of $1 bills, and more than one woman has told us that she donated her eggs to get the money for breast surgery.

◗ Can I deduct breast implants as a business expense?

It depends on how you use them. Exotic dancer Cynthia Hess, better known as Chesty Love, deducted $2,088 from her taxes to cover the cost of her breast augmentation. When the IRS objected, she took her case to tax court. The judge allowed the write-off; he ruled that her enhanced breasts were necessary stage props because they were used to generate revenue at the Indiana strip club where she worked. The 1994 case made tax law history.

Are Implants Marital Assets?

According to the Bismarck Tribune, *when Erik and Traci Isaacson of North Dakota were going through a divorce in 2008, Erik demanded that the $5,500 he had spent on Traci's breast implants be counted as marital assets, which would entitle him to additional property in the breakup. The lower court said his claim was "absolute nonsense." Presiding judge Robert Wefald asked Erik's attorney, "Do you want me to have them cut out and given to Mr. Isaacson?" Erik took his claim to the North Dakota Supreme Court, which ruled against him, too. He also sought sole custody of his three children. Maybe he can ask for visitation rights for those breast implants.*

What is the fair market value of a used breast implant?

THE **BREAST THINGS** IN LIFE ARE FREE

Venezuelan politician Gustavo Rojas isn't the only sponsor of a contest for free breast implants. Radio stations in the United States and Canada have run "Breast Summer Ever" contests: Listeners are invited to submit a photo and a statement explaining why they should win. Pictures are posted on the station's website, and the public determines who is most deserving of the prize. Here are some other booby benefactors:

- For several years, the Royal Australian Navy paid for female sailors to have breast augmentation surgery. The implants weren't meant to be used as personal flotation devices in the event of an emergency. They were intended for women whose small breast size caused psychological distress that interfered with their job performance. Each breast augmentation cost $10,000. Nice use of taxpayer money.

- In 2009, the Miss California Organization paid for implants for Carrie Prejean, then Miss California, just weeks before the Miss USA competition. Prejean was later stripped of her Miss California crown because of alleged contract violations, and she was also sued by pageant officials, who wanted to be reimbursed for her $5,200 breast augmentation.

- At MyFreeImplants.com, women rely on the kindness of strangers to raise money for breast augmentation surgery. After a woman creates a profile and posts pictures online, she can interact with potential contributors. Her new friends can make a direct donation to her cause; in return, they receive messages, photos and/or videos. One woman boasted that 164 men contributed to the cost of her surgery. And you thought Facebook was fun!

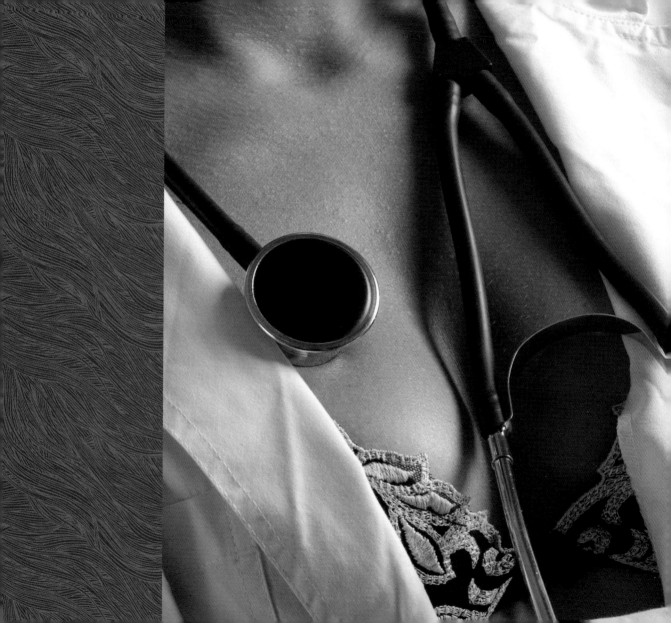

CHAPTER 6

Surgery: Ready, Set, Go

Everyone loves those before-and-after photos,
but there's no after without the in-between –
preparation for breast augmentation surgery and
the surgery itself.

Read on to get the scoop.

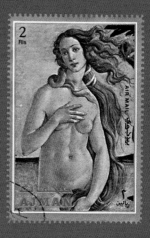

NOTE:

I perform cosmetic breast surgery in a hospital operating room, and my patients receive general anesthesia. They are completely asleep and totally unaware of their surgery. These factors, plus my preferences and those of the anesthesiologists, shape my preoperative protocol. A surgeon who operates in a surgicenter and whose patients receive local and/or intravenous (IV) sedation would likely have different answers to a number of these questions.

▶ Why do I have to get lab tests before surgery?

We want to be certain that you are in good health. Blood tests determine if you're pregnant or anemic, if your blood clots in time, and if you have an infection. If your health history warrants it, you might need additional tests, such as an electrocardiogram (EKG) or a thyroid test, for example.

▶ I know I'm not pregnant, so why do I need a pregnancy test?

In any given year, a handful of women who know they aren't pregnant are surprised by a positive pregnancy test. Because the anesthesia given during surgery and the medications prescribed for comfort afterward can affect the health of a baby, every patient gets a blood test for pregnancy as part of the presurgical testing protocol at the hospital, unless she has had a tubal ligation or a hysterectomy.

⊙⊙ Titbit: The medical term for breast augmentation is augmentation mammaplasty: "Mamma," Latin for teat, is also the root word of mammal. "Plasty" comes from the Greek word meaning formed or molded.

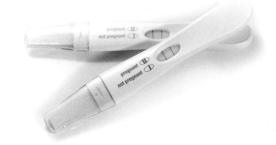

Do I need a mammogram?

Depending on your age and your family history, you may be asked to get a mammogram (an X-ray picture of the breast) before surgery. The American Cancer Society recommends mammography screenings for women 40 and older, but if a woman's mother or sister had breast cancer, we would send her for a mammogram at any age.

Do I have to quit smoking before I have surgery?

No, but I would be shirking my duty as a doctor if I didn't suggest that now would be a good time for you to stop smoking. I also know how hard it is to quit and that some of my patients have sneaked a cigarette right before or after surgery. Here are the main concerns:

Anesthesia: Both nicotine and carbon dioxide can decrease your oxygen supply. The anesthesiologist needs to know about your smoking habits; he or she might express the possibility of some respiratory risks, such as an increased chance of bronchitis after surgery. Most of my patients are young and healthy and don't have chronic obstructive lung disease, so it's less of an issue.

Healing: Nicotine causes blood vessels to narrow, which slows down the flow of blood to the tissues and can affect the healing process. This is a concern when tissue flaps with thin skin are involved, such as in facelift surgery. It could cause a problem during a breast lift or breast reduction, but it has not been a problem for my patients during a breast augmentation.

You could finance your breast augmentation through a surgical loan company, or you could quit smoking and stash your cigarette money in a cookie jar: If you smoke a pack a day and spend $5.50 per pack (the average cost around the country), in three years you would have about $6,000 (the average cost of a breast augmentation) and much healthier lungs.

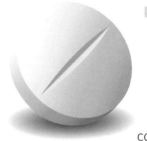

◗ If I get menstrual cramps the week before surgery, can I take Advil or Aleve?

No. Advil (a brand of ibuprofen) and Aleve (a brand of naproxen) are nonsteroidal anti-inflammatory drugs (NSAIDs), which can prolong or worsen bleeding – not by thinning your blood but by slowing down its ability to clot. Aspirin is in the same category. You could take Tylenol (a brand of acetaminophen) because it doesn't interfere with blood clotting.

We provide a list of more than 100 products that can cause bleeding problems, including drugs containing aspirin-like ingredients and some vitamins and herbal supplements. Patients are asked to stop using these products one to two weeks prior to surgery. If necessary, they can be started up again as early as four days after surgery.

◗ Can I have surgery if I have a cold?

If you were to get a cold the week before surgery, we would ask you to schedule an appointment with your family doctor to determine if it's a common cold, which is viral in nature, or if your symptoms are being caused by a bacterial infection. We are particularly concerned about bacterial infections, such as in your sinuses, chest, or even your tooth, because the bacteria could migrate

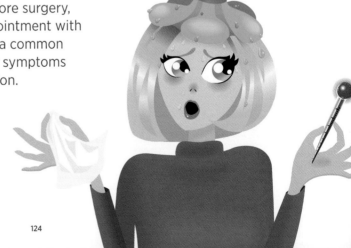

to your breast implants. You can't have surgery until the infection has been treated and your blood count is normal.

You should be infection-free for approximately two weeks before you proceed with surgery. If you wake up with a sore throat on the day of surgery – and your repeat blood test does not indicate an infection – it's a judgment call. We lean toward not operating because breast augmentation is elective surgery, and there's no reason to put you at risk.

▶ Can I have a glass of wine the night before surgery to help me relax?

You should not drink any alcohol for 48 hours before surgery. Alcohol can increase the risk of complications and slow down the recovery process. However, when you are no longer taking narcotics and muscle relaxants and have had your first postoperative visit, feel free to pop open a bottle of champagne and celebrate.

▶ Can I eat breakfast before I come to the hospital?

No. If you are having IV sedation or general anesthesia, it's crucial that you have nothing to drink, eat or chew (including gum) after midnight prior to your surgery. If you don't follow these instructions, the anesthesiologist will cancel your surgery.

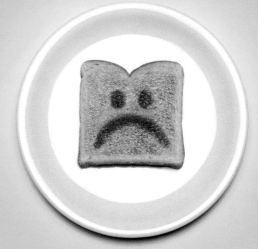

❱ If I did cocaine last night, can I have surgery?

No. The anesthesia team would cancel surgery because cocaine and other stimulants increase the irritability of the heart muscle. If your heart were to develop an irregularity during surgery, it might be difficult to control it.

During preadmission testing, patients are asked if they use recreational drugs and with what frequency. If your answer raises concern, the anesthesia team might ask you again the morning of surgery. It's essential that you tell the truth. Your answers are confidential and will not be disclosed to anyone.

Cocaine With Your Surgery

In the late 1800s and early 1900s, cocaine had an essential role in the operating room. It was used as a local anesthetic for eye surgery. It was also injected into nerves or the spine to numb specific areas. Cocaine was used in patent medicines because of its pain-relief and stimulant properties. Once its addictive properties became known, scientists developed synthetic substitutes; one of the first was Novocain.

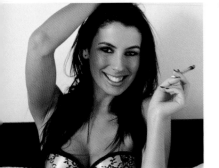

❱ If I smoked weed this morning, can I have surgery?

Maybe. The anesthesia team makes the final decision on whether or not it's safe to have surgery, so there are no guarantees. Smoking marijuana would probably be considered much like smoking cigarettes. (See page 123.)

What's Your Favorite Number?

When British author and math wizard Alex Bellos conducted a survey of favorite numbers, he discovered that 7 had the most fans. He wasn't surprised. "In Western culture, the number 7 is considered lucky, and 7 is unusual in the English language as the only digit that requires two syllables. That makes it pretty darn special," he explained.

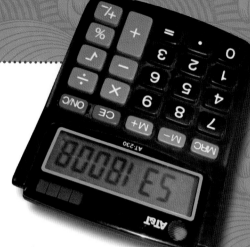

He was surprised by the number of English speakers who picked 5,318,008 as a favorite. The reason: When these digits are entered into a calculator and the calculator is turned upside down, it spells BOOBIES. There's no need to feel left out if you live in Finland or Brazil: Just enter 715,517 to spell TISSIT, Finnish for "boobies," or 50,135 to spell SEIOS, Portuguese for "breasts."

If your friends complain that you are acting like a third-grader, just tell them that you are practicing your "beghilos," the technical term for "calculator spelling."

THE OTHER BOOBIES:

The blue-footed booby is a tropical seabird that lives along the Pacific coast. In breeding season, male boobies strut and show off their blue feet to entice prospective mates.

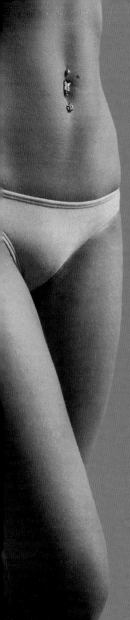

▶ Can I have surgery while I have my period?

In my experience with more than 5,000 women, surgery has never been delayed because of a menstrual cycle. There's speculation that the hormonal changes might increase the chance of bleeding in the operative field, but I have never found this to be a problem.

▶ Can I keep my underwear on during surgery?

Yes, if you are having a breast augmentation or a breast lift. If you will be under anesthesia for more than two or three hours, such as during a breast reduction, the anesthesia team might elect to insert a urinary catheter in your bladder to monitor the amount of fluids that you take in and urinate out. In that case, you would take off your underwear.

▶ Can I keep my piercings in during surgery?

Nipple rings, belly button rings, earrings, dermal anchors, and other body jewelry should be removed to avoid the risk of burns. Nonmetallic spacers can be temporarily placed in these holes to keep them open. Here's the concern: During surgery, an electrocautery is used to stop small blood vessels from bleeding. Metal body piercings could divert the electrical current from the surgical site and cause an electrical burn.

Piercings around your mouth – in your nose, lip or tongue – must be removed (and no spacers may be used) so that the jewelry doesn't end up in your airway when you get anesthesia.

◗ Do I have to take off my nail polish before surgery?

The anesthesiologist uses a pulse oximeter, a noninvasive medical device, to measure the percentage of oxygen in your blood during surgery. The device emits pulses of light; to do its job, it has to be clipped to a translucent area of the body, such as a fingernail. That's why you are asked to remove the polish from one nail. If you have acrylic nails, you don't have to remove one; the device can be clipped onto your earlobe instead.

◗ Should I bring a bra with me the day of surgery?

Each surgeon has his or her preference. I ask my patients to bring a sports bra with them. It's helpful to buy one that opens in the front. The bra is put on in the recovery room.

◗ How long can my friend stay with me before surgery?

Your support person can stay with you until you are transferred to the operating room. That means he or she can be by your side when you meet the anesthesiologist and when I mark the incision site, take pictures for you and your records, and review your postoperative medications and diet. Then you'll have to say goodbye – or ta-ta!

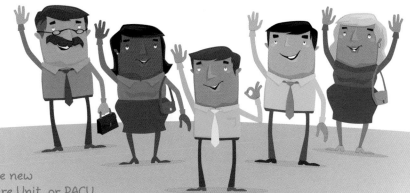

⊙⊙Titbit: The term "recovery room" has gotten a makeover. The new designation is Post-Anesthesia Care Unit, or PACU.

▶ Will the entire hospital staff see my breasts?

There won't be a crowd of onlookers. About six people are involved in your care, and all of them are professional, discreet, and interested only in helping you. Before surgery, a nurse from the Short Procedure Unit will help you get changed into a hospital gown. The operating room team includes the anesthesiologist, anesthesia nurse, circulating nurse, surgical tech and nurse assistant. Occasionally, another nurse might come in to relieve a co-worker.

Her Breasts Were Seen by Thousands

When Chinese dance coach Wang Yixuan was offered a free breast augmentation by a cosmetic surgery hospital in Beijing, she started a blog called "Flat-chested Dancer's Bosom Operation Diary." A friend filmed her operation from start to finish and posted the photographs online. In China, where maintaining dignity and avoiding embarrassment are so important, Yixuan's openness caused an Internet controversy.

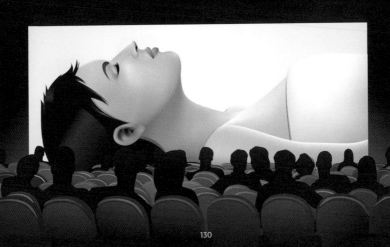

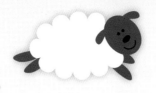

▶ Will I be completely asleep?

Yes, if you have general anesthesia. Before you go into the operating room, a nurse will put an intravenous (IV) line into a vein in your arm or your hand. Through that line, the anesthesiologist will first give you some medication to relax you; patients tell me it makes them feel as if they have had a couple of drinks. Next, you'll get a stronger medication that puts you completely to sleep. You won't know or feel anything. You'll wake up after the procedure with no memory of the surgery; some women don't remember anything until they are in the postoperative lounge.

It's Only a Movie

The 2007 crime thriller Awake *is the story of a man who is awake and aware but paralyzed during his heart transplant surgery. That's how he finds out that his friends are plotting to kill him. It's not true; it's only a movie. During surgery, your blood pressure and heart rate are continually monitored, and we can tell if you are uncomfortable – even on a subconscious level. We're not depending on you to tell us.*

▶ Will I say something to embarrass myself during surgery?

Anesthesia is not a truth serum that makes you disclose your deepest secrets. It doesn't loosen your tongue; it simply makes you relax and fall asleep. However, the last thought you have before drifting off to sleep may be the first thought you have upon awakening. One woman woke up, looked down, grabbed her breasts and said, "I have boobies!" She had a big smile on her face.

What's the difference between local anesthesia and IV sedation?

Local anesthesia is used to block sensation in a particular part of the body. During cosmetic breast surgery, the breasts are numbed with injections of a dilute analgesic like Xylocaine, similar to what's used by your dentist. If you have local anesthesia only, you'll be fully awake during surgery.

For intravenous (IV) sedation, you are given a combination of medications that produces "twilight sleep." You'll be relaxed but not unconscious. You might be able to hear what the doctor is saying and respond to a question, but afterward you will most likely not remember anything that happened during surgery.

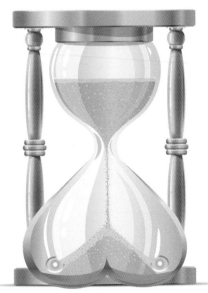

Some surgeons perform cosmetic breast surgery while the patient is under general anesthesia; others use local anesthesia, intravenous sedation, or a combination of the two.

Will I lose a lot of blood during surgery?

No. Patients generally lose less than a teaspoon of blood during breast augmentation surgery.

How long does a breast augmentation take?

It varies from surgeon to surgeon. It takes me less than one hour.

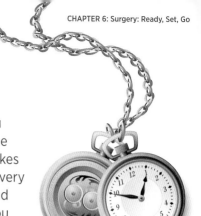

How long will I be in the hospital?

If I'm your doctor, you'll be there for six hours from the moment you check in until you leave for home. You generally have to report to the hospital 90 minutes before your scheduled surgery time. Surgery takes approximately one hour. Afterward, you'll be transferred to the recovery room, where specially trained nurses will monitor your vital signs and help you transition into a more awake and alert state. They'll give you liquids and medicine to keep you comfortable, and they'll help you put on your sports bra. You'll stay there for about two hours.

You'll spend the last hour in the postoperative lounge, where you'll get dressed, sit up, and eat some cookies or crackers. Before you're discharged, the nurses will remove your IV line and give you instructions to follow at home. Your significant other/friend can spend this last hour with you.

Do I have to have surgery in a hospital?

While some physicians perform surgery in a hospital operating room, others do office-based procedures or work in an ambulatory surgery center, sometimes called a surgicenter. These freestanding centers are equipped for emergencies and are generally affiliated with a nearby hospital, where patients with more serious problems can be transferred. In 1996, California became the first state to require accreditation for any outpatient facility that administers sedation or general anesthesia. Many other states have followed suit.

⊙⊙Titbit: Outpatient surgery, also called ambulatory surgery, does not require an overnight hospital stay. It can be performed in a surgicenter or in a hospital operating room.

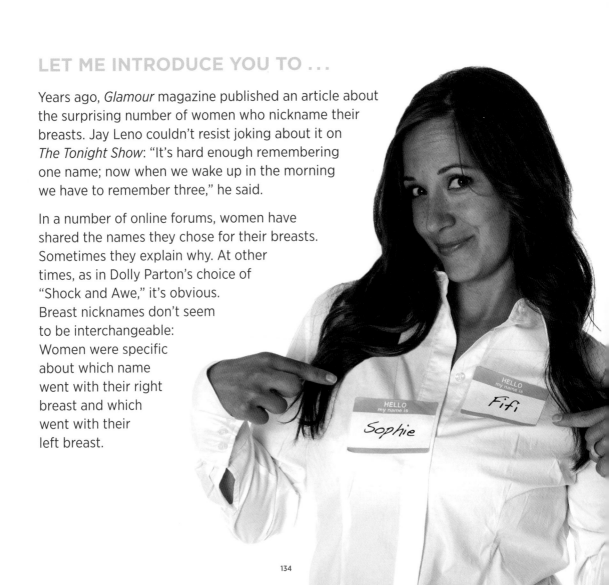

LET ME INTRODUCE YOU TO ...

Years ago, *Glamour* magazine published an article about the surprising number of women who nickname their breasts. Jay Leno couldn't resist joking about it on *The Tonight Show*: "It's hard enough remembering one name; now when we wake up in the morning we have to remember three," he said.

In a number of online forums, women have shared the names they chose for their breasts. Sometimes they explain why. At other times, as in Dolly Parton's choice of "Shock and Awe," it's obvious. Breast nicknames don't seem to be interchangeable: Women were specific about which name went with their right breast and which went with their left breast.

HERE'S A SAMPLING OF SOME OF OUR FAVORITES:

- License and Registration

- Lucy and Ethel

- Siegfried and Roy

- Gin and Tonic

- Thelma and Louise

- Cheech and Chong

- These Are Not and My Eyes, Buster

- Bogie and Bacall: "Old style, but still a classic pair."

- Tutti and Frutti: "I named them on a trip to a Caribbean island."

- Hoss (left) and Little Joe (right): "I'm slightly larger on the left side."

- Paris and Nicole

- Gladys and Ethel: "They have old lady names now. Maybe one day they will graduate to stripper names."

- Ben and Jerry: "Once I started eating more ice cream, they started growing, so I figured it was only right. Right now Jerry is being a little poop and not staying in place."

- Bill and Ted: "... because they have excellent adventures."

- Ariel and Jasmine: "That's how my boyfriend refers to them. I have no idea why he named them after Disney princesses."

- Handel and Mozart

- Chip and Dale: "... because I was motioning at the picture of Chip and Dale on my sweatshirt and my friend thought I was talking about my boobs."

- "My boyfriend has a multitude of nicknames for them. Mostly they're made-up superheroes."

- Naughty and Nice: "because one nipple is pierced and the other isn't. Variety is the spice of life, right?"

- Dyan and Pachelbel: "Two great canons."

- Tweety and Sylvester

- Itty and Bitty

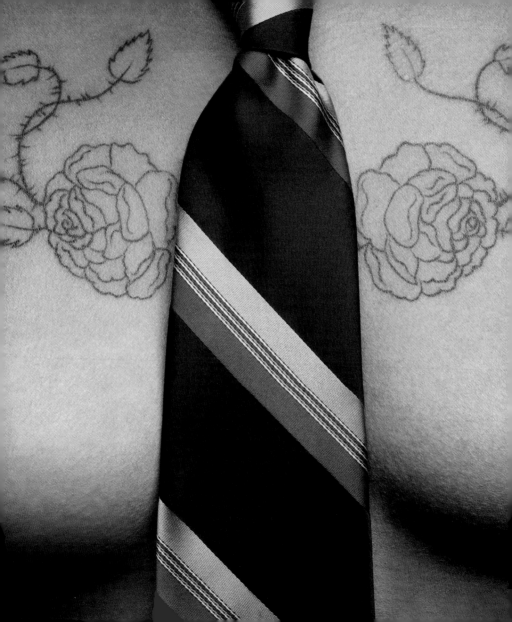

CHAPTER 7

Recovery: Is That Normal?

"From small beginnings come great things." – author unknown

"Are we there yet?" Remember asking your parents that question from the back seat of the car on a long summer trip? It's not much different from the questions patients ask after cosmetic breast surgery, when they are anxious to get to the beach: "How soon can I...?" When will they...?" "Is it normal for...?" Like your parents told you: "It won't be too long."

Here's what you can expect to see on the ride.

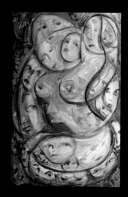

NOTE: *The information contained in this chapter is what I tell my patients to do and to expect the first week after breast augmentation surgery and in the weeks that follow. This protocol is based on my experience and my surgical approach: The majority of my patients have saline implants. I place the implants beneath the pectoral muscle through an inframammary incision (in the crease of the breast). Surgery is performed in a hospital operating room under general anesthesia.*

Each doctor has his or her own surgical approach, suturing technique, and specific postoperative protocol, and it might vary greatly from what you read here. It is imperative that you follow your doctor's instructions.

WEEK ONE

Can I wear a seat belt on the ride home?

You can and you should. A seat belt won't harm your implants. I have had patients who buckled up and rode home the eight-plus hours from Philadelphia to Central Ohio right after surgery. For comfort, some have placed a small square or rectangular pillow between their chest and the upper-body seat belt.

Should I put heat or ice on my breasts when I get home?

After breast augmentation surgery, an ice pack or a bag of frozen peas can provide some comfort. Ice, which helps reduce swelling, is best for the first 48 hours after surgery. After that, heat is better for discomfort and aches, like a backache, because it brings more blood to the area and helps relieve pain and spasms.

When can I take a shower or bath?

You can take a shower the day after surgery, but you should wait until the third week to take a bath. If you soak in a tub, the water could penetrate the incision and cause an infection, whereas the shower water runs off the incision and doesn't soak into it.

How much pain will I have?

Women usually describe the feeling as discomfort, not pain. Those who have had children say they feel as they did when their breasts were fully engorged with milk after childbirth. Women who haven't had children describe the feeling as tightness, burning or pressure. The discomfort usually starts to ease up on the fourth day after surgery. Until then, you can take the medications that are prescribed to make you comfortable during the recovery period.

Will I be able to brush my hair and my teeth myself?

Yes. You will be able to move your arms after breast augmentation surgery although you might have some discomfort or stiffness when doing so.

⊙⊙Titbit: For your substitute ice bag, pick a frozen vegetable that you don't intend to eat. Experts say that refreezing a thawed vegetable diminishes its flavor, texture and nutritional value.

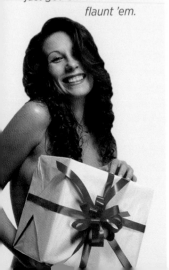

When can I pick up my baby?

For the first few days, you will need to depend on someone else to lift your baby. Beginning on Day 3 (if you had surgery on Monday, Day 3 is Thursday), you can lift your baby – when necessary – into and out of a crib, high chair or car seat. This restriction is to ensure your comfort and minimize the risk of bleeding around the implants. If I could, I would make you wait longer, but I understand that most women can't depend on someone else to help them for an entire week. You should not carry your child around all day until a couple of weeks after surgery.

Do I have to stay in bed for a few days?

No, but after surgery you do need time to rest and heal, and you should take it easy for one week. Listen to your body and to me – not to the voice in your head that tells you the laundry needs to be done now. Patients sometimes call me on Day 2 and ask why their breasts feel so sore. When I ask what they did, they tell me they vacuumed their entire house or carried their laundry basket up and down the stairs. After exerting themselves, they realized that they did too much too soon. Leave the vacuum cleaner in the closet for a few weeks; if you need an excuse note, I will be happy to write one for you.

Leave the car in the driveway, too. Anesthesia stays in your system for at least 24 hours after surgery, which means you'll be a little groggy. You might also be taking pain medication for the first few days. If you aren't taking any narcotics, you can probably drive as early as Day 3.

I can't sleep on my back. What am I going to do?

You don't have to sleep on your back or sit up all night after breast augmentation surgery. You can sleep any way you want from the night of surgery on, including on your stomach, if you are comfortable enough. You won't pop or displace your implants by sleeping on them; they are extremely durable.

Do I need to massage my breasts after surgery?

Most likely. Massage normally implies rubbing, but for my breast augmentation patients, it means gently pulling up the skin at the top of each breast. This action pushes the implant downward, which helps keep the bottom of the pocket around the implant open. We're relying on Newton's third law of motion: For every action, there is an equal and opposite reaction – although he probably did not have this in mind. In time, when the skin stretches and the muscles relax, there will be space for the implants to move into. Although massage may be necessary for silicone gel implants, it's more commonly done when saline implants are used.

Now That's a Housekeeping Service!

Xia Jun, CEO of a housekeeping company in Shanghai, has started a breast massage service to help new mothers boost their milk production. After completing a three-month course at the China Employment Training Technical Instruction Center, Jun became the first man in China to be officially qualified as a breast massage therapist. He intends to train his employees to massage breasts in a scientific way and to expand his business throughout the country. His fee ranges from $46-$77 an hour. Does the price increase with cup size? Just wondering.

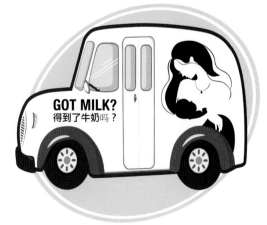

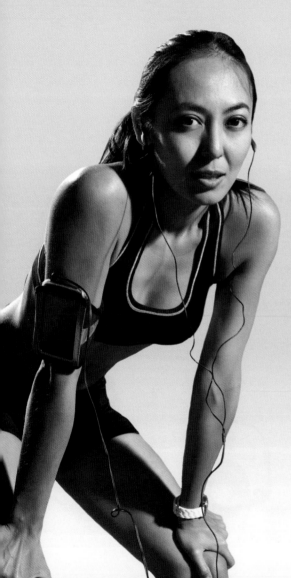

▶ How long do I have to stay wrapped up with an Ace bandage?

Some plastic surgeons wrap their breast augmentation patients with an elastic bandage after surgery, and women may be told to wear it for several weeks. I rarely use elastic bandages. I prefer to have patients do the massage as described on page 141.

▶ Will my breasts swell together if I don't keep a rolled-up Ace bandage between them after surgery?

No. You would only need to do this if you had surgery to correct symmastia (a uniboob), which can occur when the tissues in the cleavage area are overdissected. After corrective surgery, you would need to keep pressure on the cleavage area while it heals. You might be directed to use an Ace bandage and wear a compression garment like the Thongbra, which was designed just for this purpose.

▶ What bra should I wear after surgery?

Generally, my patients wear a sports bra day and night the first week after surgery, except for when they take a shower. The band at the bottom of the bra helps to re-establish the crease under the breast.

▶ What can I put on my incision – and when?

Skin likes moisture, and it's a good idea to keep the incision and the area around it moist. For the first week after surgery, it's best to use a topical antibiotic ointment. For the next five weeks, you can use any moisturizer that is gentle and unscented. After six weeks, anything goes. I prefer that patients wait until this point before considering the use of a scar cream.

No More Bouncing Breasts

In the late 1970s, a fitness craze swept the United States, and women needed a way to keep their bouncing breasts in check as they jogged or worked out. Lisa Lindahl and Hinda Miller, both avid runners, had an idea. They cut up a pair of jockstraps and sewed them together to construct the first sports bra. Their Jogbra was a huge success. Thirteen years later, Lindahl and Miller sold their company to Playtex, an international women's apparel manufacturer. Today their Jogbra has a place of honor in the collections of the Smithsonian and the Metropolitan Museum of Art.

⊙⊙Titbit: Want to learn to build a better bra? Then consider enrolling in Hong Kong Polytechnic University's degree program in Intimate Apparel, which promises students a "supportive" learning environment. Courses include Practical Bra Construction and Bra Cup Moulding.

Ode to the Onion

While onions might make you cry, they could make your scar happy because the chemical compounds in them are believed to have anti-inflammatory properties. That's what companies are banking on when they use onion extract in their topical scar creams. The extract is listed on the label as Allium cepa.

Thank goodness someone figured out how to make onion extract, or you might be tying onions around your breasts: In Malta, when someone is bitten by a sea urchin, one-half of a baked onion is tied to his or her wound. The Maltese also consider the onion to be an aphrodisiac, but that's another story.

When do I get my stitches out?

Some doctors close the incision with stitches on the outside, which are usually removed five to seven days after surgery. Instead of using external stitches, I put a layer of stitches just beneath the skin edge and then place an adhesive strip over the incision. There are no stitches to be removed; in my opinion, this allows for better healing.

If my incision opens, will my implants fall out?

The likelihood of your incision opening is extremely low because it is closed with multiple layers of stitches that take months to dissolve. In the rare case of an infection that prevents healing, for example, the implant would be too big to fall out through the incision. That's why we don't include an easy reinstallation kit in your postoperative package.

When can I have sex?

You should abstain for a full week. Sexual activity could raise your blood pressure and cause bleeding around the implants. At the first postoperative visit, I will examine you to make sure you are healing well before I give you the go-ahead.

After my augmentation, can I let my boyfriend touch my breasts?

Your breasts may look like a masterpiece, but there's no need to hang a "Please Don't Touch the Art" sign on them. Breast augmentation is an investment that you can enjoy. There's no need for a "You Break It, You Buy It" sign either. Your breast implants aren't fragile.

Will my partner be able to squeeze my breasts or be a little rough without popping the implants?

It's best to wait at least three weeks before "being a little rough"; then be sure to listen to your body. You might feel sore or uncomfortable, but it won't harm your implants – unless your partner can squeeze your breasts with significantly more force than a mammogram does.

"No Mufky-Fufky"

That's how one of the senior surgeons referred to sex years ago when we made rounds in the hospital. "No mufky-fufky," he would tell his patients after surgery, warning them not to get "too frisky." That was a new one for me!

When can I go back to work?

It depends on what your job entails. More than 90 percent of my patients go back to work on the fifth day after surgery if they work in an office setting. Women who must use their arms to lift, push or pull (such as nurses, hairstylists or waitresses) normally return to work toward the end of the second week, around the 14th day after surgery. Although they may experience a little discomfort, they manage.

Housework counts as work, too. If your household activities include lifting laundry baskets and pushing a heavy vacuum, you should put off these chores until the 14th day as well. My preference is for women to wait until the 21st day to resume activities that involve lifting, pushing or pulling. At this point, most soreness is gone.

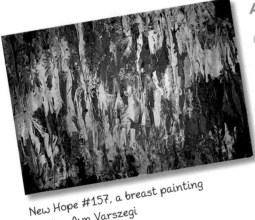

New Hope #157, a breast painting by Kira Ayn Varszegi

After Surgery, You Could Put *Them* to Work

Connecticut artist Kira Ayn Varszegi has given new meaning to the phrase "breast stroke." Since 2001 she's been covering her 38DD breasts in paint and pressing them against canvases to produce what she calls "ridiculously beautiful abstract things created in unorthodox ways." You can see her impressive body of work at TurtleKiss.com.

At the Buttercups Ceramic Studio in County Durham, England, women have redefined "breast plate." They are dipping their breasts in paint and imprinting them on plates to make images of cherries, bumblebees, pandas and Christmas puddings.

IS THAT NORMAL?

◗ Why is my left breast more tender than my right?

From the first day of surgery on, patients commonly say that one breast is more tender than the other, and they are concerned that something is wrong. This is absolutely normal and happens to all patients. Breast augmentation is actually two separate surgeries (one on the left side and one on the right side), so it's no surprise that each side heals at a different rate and with a different sensitivity from the other.

◗ Am I crazy? I think I hear my implants sloshing around.

It's perfectly normal. Women hear their implants slosh, gurgle, squeak, crackle, and even "talk" to them. It's not the implants that are making noise; the sounds are coming from antibiotic fluids that were used during surgery and/or from the air that has built up in the pocket around the implant. As your body absorbs the fluid and the air bubbles, the sounds disappear – usually three to five weeks after surgery.

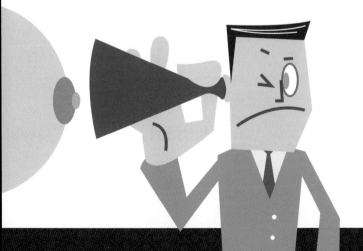

My right breast looks bigger. Did you get mixed up and put more saline in that one?

There's no way this can happen. Here's the process:

- The left and right implant fill volumes (ccs) are recorded in your office chart. You review the chart and give your approval.

- I show this chart to the OR team – the circulating nurse, surgical tech and nurse assistant – and review the plan with them.

- The left and right implant fill volumes (ccs) are written on the board in the operating room.

- Each time I put a full syringe of saline solution (50 ccs) into the implant through the valve, all four of us count aloud. One person records it on paper until we reach the goal.

What's the likelihood of four people miscounting or mixing up right and left? **Zero.**

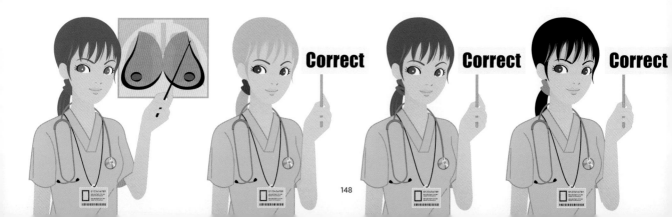

▌ My nipples are so sensitive they hurt. What's going on?

Sometimes the nerve to the nipple is temporarily stretched during surgery. While it's healing, there may be a short-term, annoying increase in sensation for about six weeks before the nerve returns to normal. For most women, there is no permanent increase, decrease, or loss of nipple sensation.

▌ Is it normal for my implants to be so high?

It is normal, particularly if you have saline implants that were placed under the muscle. The pectoral muscle presses the implant flat, as your hand would compress a sponge ball or a balloon, and the implant needs a place to go. It is limited on three sides by the breastbone and the outside edges and bottom of the breast, so it moves toward the area of least resistance: the collarbone and the armpit.

As the skin stretches and the muscles relax, the implants move down and out slowly – about 1 percent a day. It'll be about six weeks before they even begin to settle down, but they'll be close to 80 percent settled at three months. Watching their progress is like watching your hair grow. You don't see a difference in your hair growth daily, but all of a sudden you need a haircut. Give yourself a few months before making a judgment about your surgical results.

Silicone gel implants start out lower than saline implants, closer to their final position. That's because more muscle is released to create a bigger space for the prefilled gel implants; as a result, they are less compressed right after surgery.

I've Got Boobies!

"As I reflect back on old photos, I cannot imagine the old self-conscious flat-chested me wearing my strapless, sweetheart neckline gown. I can't thank you enough for giving me the chance to choose any gown I wanted for my wedding day."

"Every summer, when I'm in my non-padded bikini top, I think of and silently thank you for the beautiful job you did on my breast augmentation."

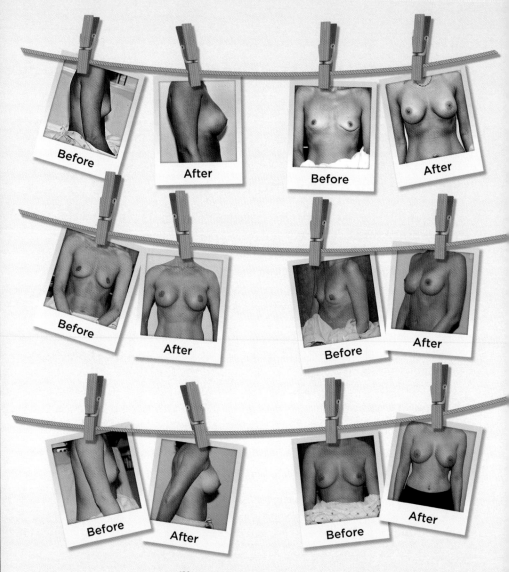

Before

After

Before

After

Before

After

Before

After

Before

After

Before

After

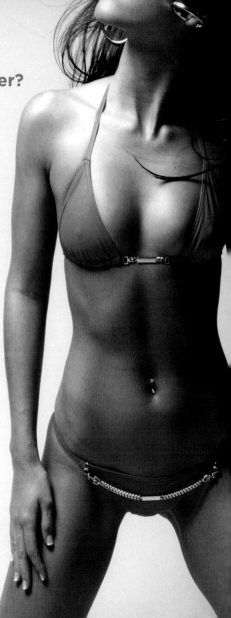

▶ Why does one breast look higher than the other?

Right after surgery is too soon to be evaluating implant size and position. Remember that one breast often heals at a different rate from the other, and one breast may be more swollen. Three months after surgery, you will be about 80 percent healed, but it can take up to nine months for settling and healing to be fully complete.

▶ If the implants have to move down into place, how do they know where to stop? Could they drop to my stomach?

Implants don't come with a built-in GPS system programmed with a final destination. They don't need one. After three weeks, a normal capsule or lining starts to form around the implants, so they can't get lost: There's no other place for them to go. Plus, there's a natural limit to the amount the skin can stretch.

▶ What if my implants don't drop down?

After six months, if one or both implants don't come down, a minor surgical revision can be done to allow the implant to fill out the lower breast tissue. On average, this problem occurs in up to 5 percent of breast augmentations. Massage done in the first few months after breast augmentation surgery might help reduce the need for revision.

Is it normal for my breasts to be this hard?

Yes. Because the muscle flattens the implants, the implants have limited space in which to move right after surgery, and they feel hard. They will feel softer over time as the muscle relaxes and the skin stretches.

Is it normal for my implants to move up during the day and back down at night?

It could happen. If you are active during the day, the pectoral muscle might tighten and push up your implants. At night, if you are relaxed, the muscle might relax, too, allowing the implants to move down a bit.

Should I be able to feel my breast implants through my skin?

It's possible – and common – to feel the implants on the sides and underneath the breasts where there is little or no muscle coverage.

Why do my breasts feel heavy?

After augmentation surgery, some women describe their breasts as feeling heavy or full. One woman said it felt as if there were two aliens on her chest. Women who have breastfed compare it to how they felt in the mornings when their breasts were full and their baby hadn't yet nursed.

The actual weight of the implants is minimal, but breasts do feel heavy as the skin stretches and the muscles heal. The good news is that at about five weeks after surgery, women say they are accustomed to the weight of their new breasts and can't remember how they felt without implants. It's not much different from adjusting to new glasses or contact lenses.

HOW SOON CAN I ...

⟩ How soon can I go back to the gym?

It depends on what you want to do there. Three weeks after surgery, it's OK for you to do aerobic activity (treadmill, stationary bike, etc.), running and lower-body weight training. Women are usually comfortable doing arm exercises (upper-body weights) starting about six weeks after surgery.

Dancing Implants

If your implants were placed under the muscle, they might move up and down when you flex your pecs. They'll dance, so to speak. It might be apparent at the gym, and it could come in handy as a party trick. You don't have to quit doing bench presses and push-ups. There's no way you could compress the implants enough to damage them.

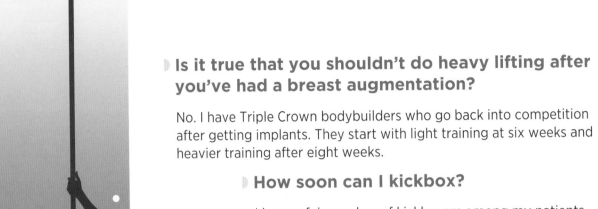

Is it true that you shouldn't do heavy lifting after you've had a breast augmentation?

No. I have Triple Crown bodybuilders who go back into competition after getting implants. They start with light training at six weeks and heavier training after eight weeks.

How soon can I kickbox?

I have a fair number of kickboxers among my patients, and they seem to be comfortable getting back to their sport at around six weeks after surgery. None of their implants has deflated.

How soon can I get back to using the pole or dancing topless?

Patients tell me that they can "prance" as early as 7 to 10 days after surgery, but it takes about three weeks until they are comfortable again with the pole.

A Word You Should Know

"Tittup" is a verb that means to prance or strut, often in an exaggerated or affected way. Let's use it in a sentence: "The overdressed women tittuped past us on their way to the club." It's one of the words that the young contestants were asked to spell in The 25th Annual Putnam County Spelling Bee, *a Tony Award-winning musical. It was not on my sixth grade vocabulary list.*

When do I have to see the doctor again?

Patients are scheduled for postoperative appointments at one week, three weeks and three months. They are asked to return at nine months, too, if possible. At that point, they are officially discharged from my care, but I tell them that we are BBF – Bosom Buddies Forever. They can call me at any time.

How soon can I wear my bulletproof vest?

More than a dozen of my patients are policewomen, and this question is important to them. The answer is that they can put their vests back on three weeks after surgery. When they come to the office for their checkups on their way to or from work, they have to take off their gun to change into an examination gown. That's one more reason why I do my best to make my patients happy!

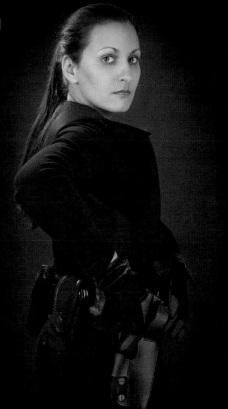

Natural Weapons

Busty Heart, aka Susan Sykes, a stripper and strip club owner, appeared on America's Got Talent *in 2008. Her gift? Crushing objects, such as soda cans, wooden boards and watermelons, with her breasts, which weigh about 20 pounds each.*

❱ When can I go in a hot tub or swimming pool?

It is wise to wait at least three weeks. At that time, the incision will be healed enough so that water won't penetrate it and possibly cause an infection.

❱ When should I go shopping for new bras?

It's best to wait at least eight weeks before making a major investment in new bras. It takes that long for your augmented breasts to begin to settle into their new size and shape. At that time, you will be able to more accurately determine your postoperative size and get a truer fit.

❱ Will I ever be able to go to the chiropractor again?

Yes, and you will be able to lie on your stomach. It's best to wait about five weeks before you schedule an appointment so as to avoid any discomfort. Don't worry about the implants popping; it's not likely that the chiropractor could exert enough force to do that.

❱ When can I go back to the tanning salon?

You can go tanning as early as three weeks after surgery. Be sure to protect your incisions with sunscreen that has a sun protection factor (SPF) of 15 or higher. Ultraviolet light, whether from the tanning bed or the sun at the beach, can make a scar redder for a longer period of time.

Unsnap, Separate the Cups, and Inhale

Your bra can probably convert from strapless to backless, but can it save your life? Dr. Elena Bodnar invented a bra that can do just that. The sexy, red Emergency Bra can be separated into two face masks that filter out harmful airborne particles. She came up with the idea when, as a young doctor, she witnessed the horror of the Chernobyl nuclear disaster.

In her acceptance speech for the 2009 Ig Nobel Public Health Prize, which recognizes "improbable research that makes people laugh and then think," Bodnar said, "Ladies and gentlemen, isn't it wonderful that women have two breasts, not just one? We can save not only our own life, but also the life of a man of our choice next to us."

Saved by Her Sports Bra

June 2008 - Jessica Bruinsma, 24, of Colorado Springs, was hiking in the Bavarian Alps when bad weather set in. She lost her way, fell 18 feet onto a rocky ledge, and was stranded. Jessica was resourceful. She attached her sports bra to a cable used to haul timber. The cable was in reach only because the system was broken, but when it was repaired three days later, her bra arrived at the base and caught the attention of a lumberjack. He had heard about a missing hiker, and he called mountain rescue. Seventy hours after her ordeal began, Jessica was lifted to safety. Now that's an emergency bra!

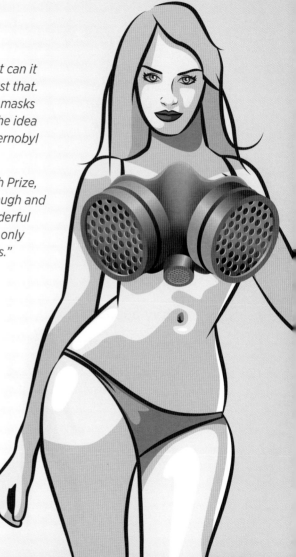

TALKING BREASTS

Fashion reporter Suzy Menkes carefully chose these ladylike words to describe breasts in her article titled "Asset Management," which appeared in *The New York Times* in August 2010:

- bust
- bustline
- chests
- cleavage
- curves
- curvy bodices
- curvy silhouette
- figure
- ripe fruit

- rounded bosoms
- rounded contours
- twin peaks
- voluptuousness

- womanly shape
- womanliness
- upper body

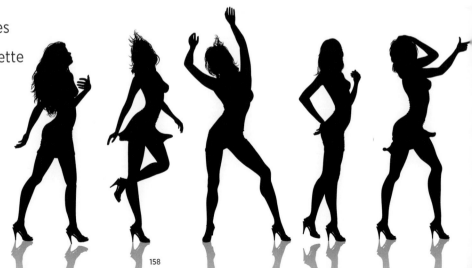

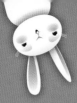

"What do you call your boobs nickname-wise?" When Dance.net posted this question on its website, its readers offered the following list of words – less classy but more colorful than Suzy Menkes' terminology.

- bazoombas
- bitties
- boobies
- breasticles
- chesticles
- jubblies
- jug-a-lugs
- knockers
- mommybops
- sack of angry rabbits
- ta-tas

- tits
- the girls
- the toddlers
- the twins
- womanly protuberances

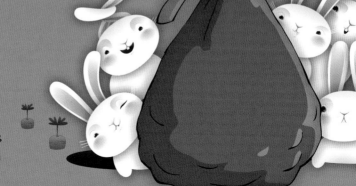

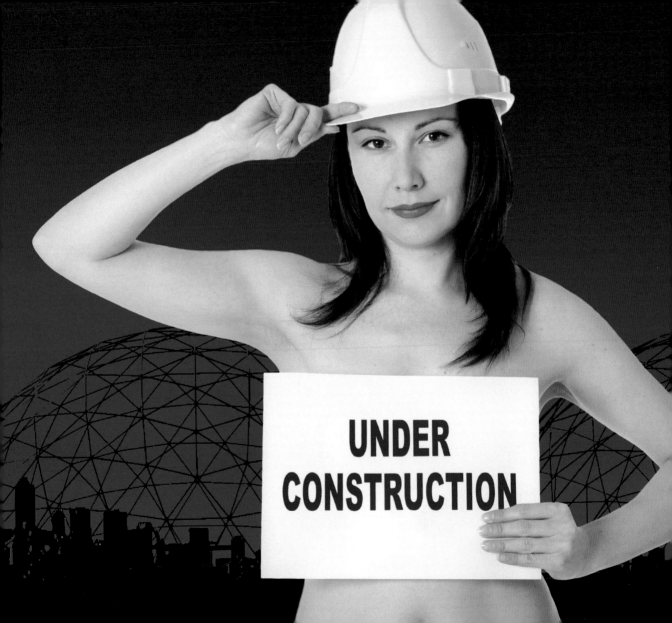

UNDER
CONSTRUCTION

Chapter 8

The Three Rs:
Raise, Reduce, Replace

Mother Nature and Father Time
have their own agendas,
but that doesn't stop us from trying to fool them.

Each year in the United States,
more than 100,000 women have surgery
to lift up breasts that have drooped
while almost as many have surgery
to reduce the size and weight of breasts
that have grown too large for their liking.

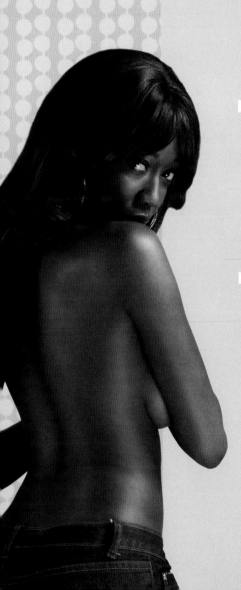

RAISE THEM: BREAST LIFTS

▶ Why do I have saggy breasts? I'm only 19.

It's not uncommon for teens to have droopy breasts. Some girls say that they were "born with saggy breasts" or that they "just developed this way." Breasts can start drooping at any age depending on your genes, the elasticity of your skin, and if you've lost a significant amount of weight. If the skin doesn't retract when some of the fat disappears from your breasts, you could be left with saggy or empty-looking breasts.

▶ I used to be perky until I breastfed my children. What happened?

When you are pregnant, the developing placenta stimulates the release of hormones, causing your milk glands – and your breasts – to grow and swell. This rapid growth can also cause the skin to stretch. When the milk is gone, some women are left with less breast volume and/or droopiness. The same thing happens as women age: The skin naturally loses its elasticity, and breasts lose their shape and firmness.

☉☉Titbit: A study in the *Aesthetic Surgery Journal* identified the following risk factors for an increased degree of breast sagging: body mass index (BMI), the number of pregnancies, a larger pre-pregnancy bra size, smoking history and age. Breastfeeding itself was not found to be a risk factor.

If I needed one, what would a breast lift do for me?

A breast lift, or mastopexy, would raise and firm your breasts, giving them a more youthful look. The surgeon accomplishes this by moving the nipples to a higher position, removing excess skin, and then reshaping the breasts.

How long after giving birth should I wait before getting a breast lift?

To know your true post-pregnancy breast size, it's best to wait at least six months from the time you give birth or from the time you stop breastfeeding, whichever is later.

If my breasts are just a little bit saggy, will implants lift them?

Implants only make you fuller; they do not lift your breasts, but they can create the illusion of a lift. As the implant fills out the upper portion of the breast, it also fills out the lower portion, which makes it appear as if the nipple is located higher on the breast.

If implants are placed behind moderately to severely droopy breasts that have not been lifted, it could give the impression that you have four breasts: the implants up high and your own breasts down low.

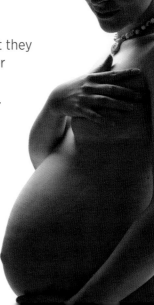

How saggy is saggy enough to need a breast lift?

Try this "pencil test" to see if you would benefit from a breast lift: Place a pencil horizontally along the crease under your breast, where your bra band would rest. Look in the mirror. Is the position of the nipple itself (not the areola) above, at or below the pencil? If your nipple hangs below the pencil, you would need a breast lift to raise and reshape your breasts. If your nipple is at the crease, the approach is not as clear-cut; it depends on how much of a pick-me-up you are hoping for. Obviously, there are other measurements done during a consultation – without a pencil – to help determine if a breast lift is the right choice for you.

⊙⊙ Titbit: In medical lingo, ptosis is the word for a drooping body part; breast ptosis is classified as mild, moderate or severe. Hint: The "p" is psilent.

What's a lollipop lift?

It is one of several options for breast lift surgery, each of which gets its name from the shape of the scar that results. The lollipop lift is often used for women with mild to moderate droopiness. The incision encircles the areola and then runs in a straight line down to the inframammary fold. It is also called a vertical-scar mastopexy.

The lollipop lift is not the only mastopexy technique named for a sweet snack: The donut lift is commonly used for women with a small amount of breast droopiness (mild ptosis). An incision is made around the areola, and

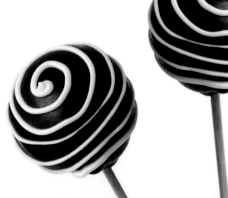

a donut-shaped segment of pigmented skin and breast skin is removed. Using a running stitch, sutures are placed along the edge of the cutout circle; when the ends of the suture are pulled, the surgical site is closed like a purse. Hence its nickname: The purse-string mastopexy.

⟩ My breasts are really droopy. What technique would you use for me?

Moderately to severely ptotic breasts are best lifted with the anchor mastopexy. The surgeon makes a circular incision around the areola, a vertical incision down to the fold under the breast, and a curved incision along this fold. After the excess skin is removed, the nipple is lifted up into its new position, and the remaining skin is sutured together to create a sling – essentially a natural support bra – that raises up the breast.

⟩ After a lift, will my breasts be bigger or smaller?

Your breasts will be the same size because only excess, stretched skin is removed during a breast lift; no breast tissue is taken away. To see how you will look after surgery, put on a good bra and gaze into the mirror. After surgery, your bare breasts might appear to be smaller than they used to be because the surgery shortened and tightened them. The change in size is just an illusion.

⊙⊙ Titbit: While a breast lift can create a nicely shaped breast, the scars from the incisions will be visible and permanent. For most women, the incisions heal to a thin line; infrequently, they may be thicker and more apparent.

Is it possible to breastfeed after breast lift surgery?

The likelihood is very strong that breast lift surgery won't affect your ability to breastfeed because your milk ducts, which run from the mammary glands to the nipple, are not disturbed. Only skin from the perimeter of the areola is removed, and there are no milk ducts there.

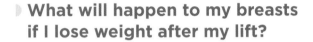

What will happen to my breasts if I lose weight after my lift?

For the most part, your breasts are made up of fatty tissue, so they might get smaller and droopier if you lose 10 percent or more of your body weight.

How long does a breast lift last?

A breast lift has long-lasting results. As you age, the newly positioned nipple and areola will generally stay above the inframammary fold. However, future pregnancies or significant weight changes can undo some of the improvement and cause your breasts to sag again.

"My husband said, 'Show me your boobs,' and I had to pull up my skirt, so it was time to get them done!" – Dolly Parton

Cosmetic Breast Surgery Around the World

Twelve of the 16 cast members on Real Housewives of New Jersey, Atlanta *and* Orange County *have breast implants. But they aren't the only ones augmenting their breasts. Their sisters in Rio and Rome and Shanghai are doing it, too.*

In 2010, 1.5 million women around the world had breast augmentation surgery, while another 550,000 had breast reductions and 540,000 had lifts, according to the International Society of Aesthetic Plastic Surgery.

Here are the top five countries for each procedure:

AUGMENTATION	LIFT	REDUCTION
U.S.	U.S.	U.S.
Brazil	Brazil	Brazil
Mexico	Mexico	China
Italy	Italy	Italy
China*	China*	India

* Colombia, France, India and Japan came in close behind China.

◉◉Titbit: If you live in Brazil, you can get a big boost in your cup size and your income tax return at the same time. A 2012 law allows citizens to deduct cosmetic surgical procedures, including breast augmentation, and it's retroactive to 2004.

The Ideal Breast Lift™: Getting Even

Have you ever tried to cut your hair yourself? You trim a little bit from the left side and then a little bit from the right side, using your ears as a guideline. Oops. It's not even, so you go back and forth and back and forth. Before you know it, your hair is too short.

Plastic surgeons have a similar challenge during breast lift surgery when they strive to even out your breasts. The traditional approach is to remove the skin on one side and tack it back together to see how it looks. They repeat the process on the other side and compare. If the breasts are not even, they go back and forth and back and forth, trimming skin until they get it right.

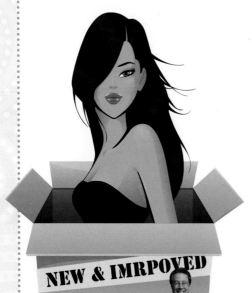

NEW & IMRPOVED
IDEAL BREAST LIFT

After years of using this approach, I had an "aha moment" and thought: What if I tacked the skin together first? Then I could see the new breast shape and symmetry before I made a single incision. It worked. With this technique, I know precisely how much skin needs to be removed. It takes the guesswork out of the procedure. It has made a significant difference for me, and I have taught the technique to surgeons around the world.

This approach is particularly useful for simultaneous augmentation mastopexy (a breast lift with implants), which is even more challenging because the surgeon has to make droopy breasts fuller by stretching the skin with implants and firmer by tightening the skin during the breast lift.

How long does breast lift surgery take?

A breast lift takes about two hours. You will be discharged and allowed to go home later the same day.

Is a breast lift painful?

Women report minimal discomfort after breast lift surgery. That's because a breast lift involves removing only loose, stretched skin. If implants are added at the same time, the skin and muscle will be stretched, which may cause a little more discomfort. By the third day, many women are comfortable enough to lift their children and to drive. More than 90 percent of my patients are back to work on the fifth day after surgery if they work in an office setting. Women whose work requires lifting, pushing or pulling usually go back to work toward the end of the second week. They might be a little sore at the end of their work day, but by Week 3, they feel pretty much back to normal.

How do I know if I need a lift and implants?

Put on your bra and look in the mirror. If you are satisfied with the size of your breasts, then a breast lift alone might be the right procedure for you. If you wish your breasts were bigger, you are probably a candidate for a breast lift and implants (an augmentation mastopexy).

Can I get a breast lift and implants at the same time?

Yes. While some doctors prefer to do two separate operations – the lift first followed a few months later by the augmentation – I perform both procedures at the same time.

(continued)

It's known as a simultaneous augmentation mastopexy. Having one surgery rather than two reduces the time that you are under anesthesia. It is a safe operation that takes about 3-1/2 hours.

❯ How much does a breast lift cost?

Prices around the country range from about $5,000 to $9,000 for breast lift surgery. If it's combined with an augmentation, expect to pay an additional $3,500 for saline implants and $4,500 for silicone. Health insurers consider a breast lift to be elective surgery and don't cover it.

Never Too Old for Nice Breasts

To date, my oldest patient was 63; she was 20 years younger than Marie Kolstad, a California woman who had a breast augmentation and lift in June 2011. She didn't tell her family about it until the day before (she didn't think they'd approve), but she did

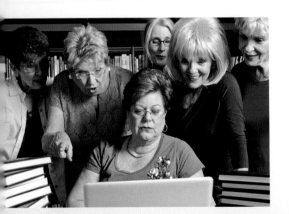

agree to do interviews afterward. At her age, she told The New York Times, "Your breasts go in one direction and your brain goes in another. Physically, I'm in good health, and I just feel like, why not take advantage of it?" During an ABC News interview, she explained, "I just wanted nice ones. I didn't want anything outlandish or out of place. Now, they are firmer and rounder."

Even if you don't want cosmetic breast surgery, you're never too old to check out the before-and-after photos online.

REDUCE THEM: BREAST REDUCTION

◗ How old do I have to be to get a breast reduction?

If you have stopped growing, which means that there have been no changes in your height, weight and breast size for two years, you would be a candidate for breast reduction surgery (reduction mammaplasty). On average, most women are finished growing by age 18.

◗ I've had back and neck pain for years. Will it go away after surgery?

Women consistently tell me that they feel an enormous amount of relief, sometimes as early as the morning after their breast reduction surgery.

Big Breasts Can Be a Pain in the Neck

Women with very large breasts often experience physical and emotional discomfort. They report a variety of medical problems, including neck, back and shoulder pain; poor posture; and numbness (a pins-and-needles feeling) in their little fingers when a nerve in their neck is pinched by the weight of their breasts. They frequently have rashes under their breasts and painful grooves in their shoulders from their bra straps. It may be difficult to exercise, particularly to run. Because their figure is out of proportion, they have trouble finding clothes that fit and flatter; it's virtually impossible to buy a dress. It's common for women to feel self-conscious about their very large breasts and the unwanted attention that they attract.

I'm on a diet. Should I wait to get a breast reduction?

Yes, because if you lose 10 percent or more of your body fat, your breasts can get smaller and droopier. The best chance of having a satisfactory long-term result is to wait until you are closer to your goal weight.

⊙⊙Titbit: It's impossible to define "very large breasts," but the women who consider breast reduction surgery often describe themselves as "top heavy." They are usually larger than a D/DD cup and their figure is out of proportion.

How many cup sizes will I lose?

The goal of breast reduction surgery is to reduce your breasts to a size and weight that are appropriate for you and more proportional for your body. It's not a one-size-fits-all approach.

There is a limit to how much tissue can be removed because there has to be enough circulation remaining to supply the nipple and areola with blood. That's why, if a woman is disproportionately large-breasted, I can sometimes reduce her size only by half, which may still leave her with a fair amount of breast tissue.

⊙⊙Titbit: In a typical breast reduction, 800-900 grams of tissue (about 2 pounds) are removed from each breast. The most I ever removed was about 7 pounds from each breast.

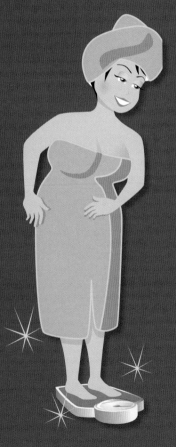

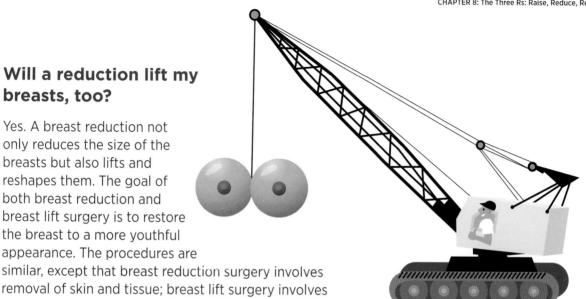

Will a reduction lift my breasts, too?

Yes. A breast reduction not only reduces the size of the breasts but also lifts and reshapes them. The goal of both breast reduction and breast lift surgery is to restore the breast to a more youthful appearance. The procedures are similar, except that breast reduction surgery involves removal of skin and tissue; breast lift surgery involves only skin.

Can you make my breasts smaller with liposuction?

Liposuction removes excess fat, so if you start out with large breasts, you could end up with a lot of loose skin and then need a lift. If your breasts are not large and not too droopy, you might be a candidate for reduction by liposuction.

What happens during breast reduction surgery?

The surgeon marks the breast to indicate the new, higher position of the nipple and the amount of breast tissue to be removed. The markings often resemble the shape of a keyhole. During the procedure, the skin and glandular tissue are excised. The nipple, which is still attached to the breast, is moved up into place.

(continued)

The breast and its envelope of skin are sewn together to restore the breast shape. In rare circumstances, when the breast is so large that circulation to the nipple cannot be maintained, the nipple is removed and grafted back on.

What does the scar look like?

The most common incision is anchorlike in shape; it goes around the nipple, extends down to the breast fold, and then runs along the breast fold.

For many women, the incision heals to a thin line; for some women, it may be thicker and more visible. During their consultation, women see photos of the incision, and they can decide if breast reduction surgery is worth the scar.

Will I be able to breastfeed after a breast reduction?

When the nipple is repositioned to a higher position, some milk ducts may be cut, which means that milk production following pregnancy could be reduced. In this case, breastfeeding might still be possible, but it may be necessary to supplement with formula.

⊙⊙ Titbit: Greek physician Paulus Aegineta is credited with the first breast reduction – in the sixth century. His patient was a man with gynecomastia (abnormal enlargement of the breasts). He recorded his experience the "Medical Compendium in Seven Books," an early medical encyclopedia.

The Devil's Cushions

In 2011, Fox News ran a story about Islamic clerics who gathered to protest padded bras. The clerics allegedly asked the Pakistani government to ban the import and sale of colorful padded bras and to make it illegal to purchase underwear in any color except white or beige. In response, the Council of Islamic Ideology proclaimed, "Padded bras are devil's cushions and he likes to rest on them" and told researchers to "try to invent a bra that makes the female chest area unnoticeable."

Fox News had been fooled: It was not a real story but a hoax that the network had picked up from a Pakistani version of The Onion. *We repeated it here because it makes us wonder: If padded bras are the "devil's cushions," what would these imaginary protestors call breast implants?*

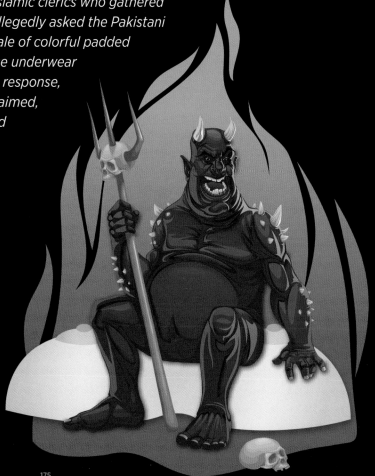

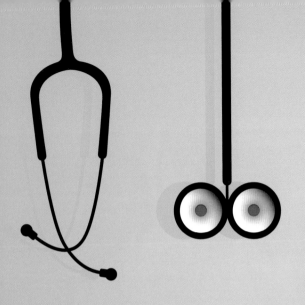

How long does the procedure take?

A breast reduction takes about three to four hours and is commonly performed under general anesthesia.

How much blood will I lose?

Very little – maybe a few tablespoons. You do not have to donate your own blood in preparation; blood transfusions are not necessary during breast reduction surgery.

Can I go home the same day after breast reduction surgery?

It varies from doctor to doctor. Because of the length of surgery and the anesthesia that's given, I like my patients to recover overnight in the hospital, so they can be observed. They are discharged in the morning. This is known as a 23-hour short stay.

Will I be uncomfortable after surgery?

Patients report minimal discomfort after breast reduction surgery. They describe a little bit of soreness underneath their breasts for a few days. Women whose work does not require lifting, pushing or pulling are generally back to work on the fifth day after surgery.

Will my health insurance pay for a breast reduction?

Health insurance often covers breast reduction surgery because of the medical problems associated with larger breasts. You can call your company before you schedule an appointment to see if coverage will be considered.

If so, you'll need to gather documentation to support your claim – a medical letter from your primary physician, X-ray reports, a list of medications, etc. Bring these to your breast reduction consultation. Your surgeon will also need to write a letter and take two photographs – a front and side view of your breasts (without your face). The whole package is sent to the medical director of your insurance company, who reviews the case and lets you know if your request is approved or denied.

If my insurance company won't cover my breast reduction, how much will I have to pay?

Prices around the country range from about $6,000 to $11,000 for breast reduction surgery.

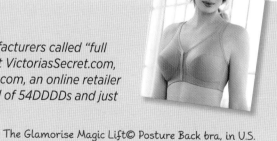

One Size Does Not Fit All

If you are one of the women who wear what the manufacturers called "full figure" bras, finding one that fits can be a challenge. At VictoriasSecret.com, 40DDD is the biggest bra available; at BareNecessities.com, an online retailer that offers more than 1,100 bras, you can find a handful of 54DDDDs and just one 56J, their largest size.

Unlike a lace demi bra, these bras do some heavy lifting: They have extra wide straps to eliminate shoulder strain, posture back support, and front closure to make it easier to put on.

The Glamorise Magic Lift© Posture Back bra, in U.S. sizes from 36B to 58J. Suggested retail price from $41.99-$43.99. Available by mail order catalog and online. For information, go to glamorise.com.

REPLACE THEM: WHEN IMPLANTS RUPTURE

About 1-3 percent of the 300,000-plus women in the United States who have a breast augmentation each year eventually have surgery to replace implants that have ruptured or deflated.

▷ What happens when a saline implant breaks?

When the implant shell tears, the saline solution leaks out quickly, usually within a few hours, sometimes in a couple of days. The implant deflates like a balloon, and the breast generally returns to its original size. Your body absorbs the saline and then you urinate it out. The saline cannot harm you: It's the same concentration as the salt water that makes up about 60 percent of the human body.

▷ What happens when a silicone gel implant breaks?

When the implant shell tears, the cohesive silicone gel inside sticks together and is unlikely to leak. You might not notice a change in breast volume or have symptoms, which is why it's called a "silent rupture." There could be no problem, or the ruptured implant could irritate the surrounding healthy tissue and cause pain, hardness or capsular contraction. Either way, the implant needs to be replaced. To check silicone gel implants for rupture, the FDA currently recommends an MRI three years after surgery and every two years thereafter. This is not covered by health insurance.

⊙⊙ Titbit: A magnetic resonance imaging (MRI) scanner uses strong magnets and a radio frequency pulse to help diagnose everything from multiple sclerosis to cancer. While a basic X-ray primarily shows the condition of bones, an MRI scan takes detailed pictures of organs and muscles as well.

If my implant deflates, how much will it cost to have it replaced?

Both silicone gel and saline implants come with a lifetime product replacement policy, which means that the manufacturer will provide a replacement implant at no cost. The implant that is not deflated can be replaced for free at the same time.

Manufacturers offer a limited warranty that is valid for 10 years from the date of initial surgery. It covers most out-of-pocket expenses for surgical fees, the operating room and anesthesia. The amount of financial assistance varies with the type of implant, the manufacturer, and whether you opt to purchase an extended warranty.

How do you replace a deflated implant?

The deflated or ruptured implant is removed, and a new implant is inserted through the original incision. Many women choose to have both the deflated implant and the intact one replaced at the same time; some also choose to go a little smaller or a little bigger, if possible.

The recuperation is easier the second time around because the pocket has already been made, and the skin doesn't have to stretch to accommodate the implant. The new implant needs only a few weeks to settle back into place; you won't have to wait as long as you did after your initial surgery.

◉◉ *Titbit: When a saline implant breaks, most women call right away because they are unhappy that they are lopsided, but one patient waited five months to call me. She didn't remember that she had a warranty; she thought she would have to pay the full price again.*

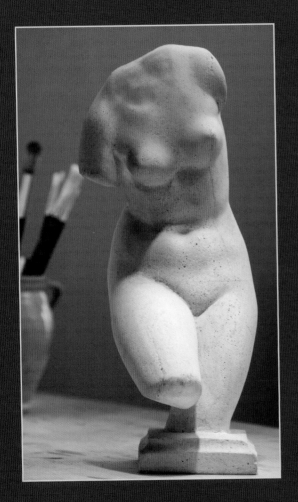

The Art of the Breast

In 2008, one lucky archaeologist discovered a small Stone Age ivory carving in a cave in southwestern Germany: At least 35,000 years old, the tiny sculpture depicted a female torso with huge breasts and wide buttocks. This "Venus of Hohle Fels," as it was named, is considered to be one of the world's oldest known examples of figurative art.

Artists and sculptors continue to put the female breast on a pedestal. They depict them as small and voluptuous, pointed and perfectly round, lifelike and idealized. Their goddesses grace Cambodian, Hindu and Egyptian temples; their Baroque beauties adorn public fountains in Italy and castle doorways in Dusseldorf. Breasts are the focal point of modern graphics, installation art, figurine ashtrays and abstract paintings.

We think it's only fitting that one well-endowed artist uses her breasts to paint abstract paintings. See page 146.

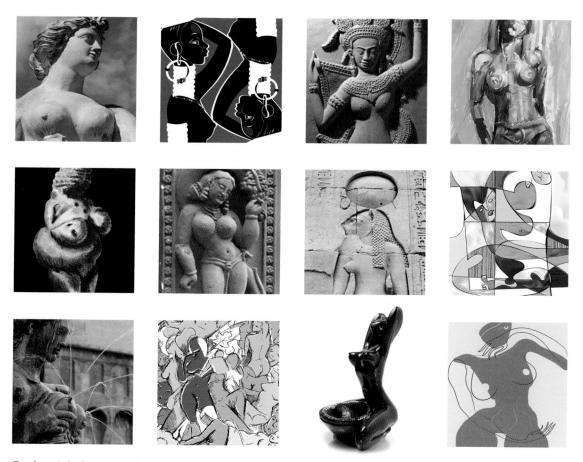

Top from left: Baroque sculpture/Dusseldorf, silkscreened poster, female divinity/Angkor Wat, abstract grunge painting.
Center from left: Venus of Willendorf illustration, Hindu temple carving, Goddess Tefnut/Temple of Horus, Cubist nude.
Bottom from left: mermaid fountain/Piazza Nettuno, Bologna, graffitti, contemporary African ashtray, line art.

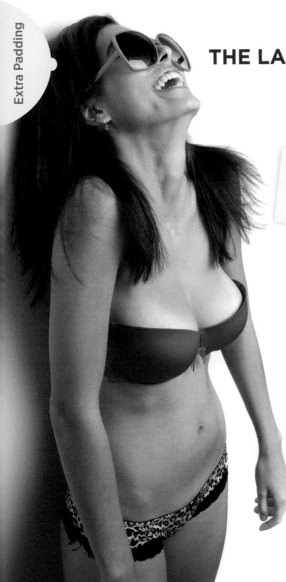

THE LAST LAUGH

"I just accepted them (my breasts) as a great accessory to every outfit."
— Jennifer Love Hewitt, named "the sexiest woman on television" in 2008 by TV Guide

"If God had intended breasts to be seen, he wouldn't have invented large woolen pullovers."
— Tracey Ullman, British comedienne

"You know it's a bad day when you put your bra on backwards and it fits better."
— anonymous

Q. What did one saggy breast say to the other saggy breast?
A. If we don't get some support soon, people will think we're nuts!
— from a Zazzle.com bumper sticker

"Your two breasts are like two fawns, twins of a gazelle, that graze among the lilies."
— Song of Songs 4:5, a biblical book of love songs, thought to be composed by King Solomon

"If life gives you lemons, I say stick 'em down your shirt and make your boobs look bigger."

— anonymous

"Ladies, here's a hint; if you're playing against a friend who has big boobs, bring her to the net and make her hit backhand volleys. That's the hardest shot for the well-endowed."

— Billie Jean King, American tennis player who won a record 20 Wimbledon titles between 1961 and 1979

"I love Thanksgiving turkey . . . it's the only time in Los Angeles that you see natural breasts."

— Arnold Schwarzenegger, who must have had some spare time to consider this topic when he was "Governator" of California

"Reaching for the stars is like reaching for breasts. Getting there doesn't guarantee that you'll be welcome."

— anonymous

"What did the bra say to the hat? You go on ahead; I'll give these two a lift."

— Soren Lauritzen, Danish author and teacher

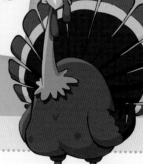

When All Is Said and Done, They're Mine!

"Three months after surgery I had a CAT scan. When the tech asked, 'Do you have implants?' I realized that I had forgotten. They felt so much a part of me." – Kristen C.

"About two months after surgery, I was driving along and reached up in a panic to make sure my implants were still there. I had totally forgotten that I had implants. That's when I knew they were mine." – Carmen S.

NOTES

CHAPTER 1:
A Tale of Two Titties

2. "senators with breasts": Claire Sargent, Democratic challenger to U.S. Sen. John McCain (Arizona, 1992), spoken at a Washington, D.C., fundraiser. See also Philip Martin, "Right Time for Sargent?" *Phoenix New Times*, Sept. 20, 1992.

5. 2010 article in the journal Pediatrics: Frank Biro et al., "Pubertal Assessment Method and Baseline Characteristics in a Mixed Longitudinal Study of Girls," *Pediatrics*, vol. 126, no. 3 (Sept. 2010), pp. 583-590.

5. In Scandinavia in the 1840s: Paul Kaplowitz, *Early Puberty in Girls: The Essential Guide to Coping with This Common Problem* (New York: Ballantine Books, 2004), pp. 64-66.

6. The U.S. Food and Drug Administration determined: "Report on the Food and Drug Administration's Review of the Safety of Recombinant Bovine Somatotropin," April 2009. To read more, www.fda/gov, search "rbGH."

7. Dressmaker Ida Rosenthal: Harold Evans, *They Made America: From the Steam Engine to the Search Engine: Two Centuries of Innovators* (New York: Little Brown and Company, 2003), pp. 309-317.

15. In Search of Miracle-Gro: Sadiq S. Moree, "Secoisolariciresinol Diglucoside: A potent multifarious bioactive phytoestrogen of flaxseed," *Research and Reviews in Biomedicine and Bio-technology (RRBB)*, vol. 2, no. 3 (2011), pp. 1-24.

17: Who's Calling?: Lynn Ray, "Ringtone That Increases Breast Size?", www.examiner.com, Sept. 10, 2010.

17. Australian women were 1 inch taller: 1999 study conducted by Newcastle University's Research Institute for Gender and Health,

commissioned by women's lingerie maker Hestia to compare the results to a survey carried out by its parent company in 1926.

25. Extra nipples: John B. Deaver and Joseph McFarland, *The Breast: Its Anomalies, Its Diseases, and Their Treatment.* (Philadelphia: P. Blakiston's Son & Co., 1917), pp. 45-101.

26. Gustavo Rojas: Andrew Cawthorne, "Politician Raffles Breast Implants," www.reuters.com, Aug. 27, 2010.

26. One elementary school's AutoCorrect: Radha Inguva, Policy Intern, National Organization for Women, "Love Your Breasts, Love Your Body," *Say It Sister*, NOW's Blog for Equality, Oct. 10, 2011.

30. Nipples at the MET: For more information about the artist, see www.jamescewart.com.

CHAPTER 2:
The ABCs of Double Ds

35. The FDA lifted its 14-year ban: "FDA Approves Silicone Gel-Filled Breast Implants After In-Depth Evaluation: Agency Requiring 10 Years of Patient Follow-Up," *FDA News Release*, Nov. 17, 2006.

37. What's That Smell?: Maged Rizkalla et al., "Trilucent Breast Implants: A 3-Year Series," *British Journal of Plastic Surgery*, vol. 54, no. 2 (2001), pp. 125-127.

39. Do implants cause breast cancer?: "What Are the Risk Factors for Breast Cancer?" American Cancer Society, www.cancer.org.

40. Another Definition of Bombshell: Rhodri Phillips, "Radicals' Deadly Booby Trap," *The Sun*, Mar. 23, 2010.

41. . . . explode at 35,000 feet: "Death On Arrival: Titty, Titty, Bang, Bang." *1000 Ways to Die: Episode 13*. Spike TV. Dec. 6, 2009.

41. MythBusters: "Cell Phone Destruction, Silicone Breasts, CD-ROM Shattering." *MythBusters: Season 1, Episode 2*. Discovery Channel. Oct. 3, 2003.

42. . . . scuba diving: Divers Alert Network (DAN) website: DAN Medical Frequently Asked Questions: www.diversalertnetwork.org/medical/faq/

44. Bulgaria: Lester Haines, "Breast Implants Save Car-Crash Bulgarian," *The Register*, Oct. 3, 2006.

44. California: Ching-Ching Ni, "Breast Implant May Have Saved Woman's Life, Doctor Says," *Los Angeles Times*, Feb. 25, 2010.

44. Jerusalem: Brit Hume, "Breast Implants Save Woman's Life," Fox News, Aug. 16, 2006.

47. Will my implants cook?: "Penny Drop, Microwave Madness, Radio Tooth Fillings." *MythBusters: Season 1, Episode 4*. Discovery Channel. Oct. 17, 2003.

49. Will a mammogram pop?: "Testing and Manufacturing of Breast Implants." Allergan, www.breastimplantanswers.com.

50. Boxing: Who Are the Boobs?: Matthew Moore, "Model Banned From Boxing Due to Breast Implants," *The Telegraph*, Feb. 16, 2009.

52. Can I be identified by my breast implants?: Cathy Kelly, "Friends Mourn Former Swimsuit Model, Bonny Doon Native," *Santa Cruz Sentinel*, Oct. 22, 2009.

53. What happens to my breast implants when I die?: Unidentified licensed funeral director and embalmer, www.answers.yahoo.com, 2007.

53. Cremation?: Deborah LeBlanc, "Ashes to Ashes - Funky Facts About Cremation," www.girlfriendbooks.blogspot.com, May 25, 2011.

53. Bosom Buddies: "Aussie Widow Puts Ashes in Breasts," *Australian News Network*, Nov. 3, 2001.

CHAPTER 3:
To B or Not to B a C or a D

60. Foxy (Great-Grand) Mama: Cosmetic Surgery National Data Bank 2011 Statistics: The American Society for Aesthetic Plastic Surgery. www.surgery.org/media/statistics.

62. Beauty Pageants, With Them: Pablo Gorondi, "Proud to Be Plastic: The 'Improved' Beauty Contest," *The Independent*, Oct. 11, 2009.

62. And Without Them: www.untamedbeauty. org.

63. I Just turned 18: "Saline-Filled Breast Implants; Silicone Gel-Filled Breast Implants." www.fda.gov/medicaldevices.

71. Can I go braless?: Amy Sohn, "Where Have All the Bras Gone," www.harpersbazaar.com, Aug. 6, 2010.

74. Was He Singing About a Uniboob?: Roger Miller (1985). The Royal Nonesuch [Rene Auberjonois]. *On Big River: The Adventures of Huckleberry Finn*. New York: Decca USA, 1990.

79. "Looking at cleavage": Jerry Seinfeld. "The Shoes." *Seinfeld: Season 4, Episode 16*. NBC. Feb. 4, 1993.

84. Trending Now in Salt Lake City: RealSelf Interest Index, 2011 Q1 site search data. www.realself.com.

CHAPTER 4:
Size Matters

91. Are You a Pear or an Apple?: 2005 study of American female body types, conducted by North Carolina State University, commissioned by Alva Products.

95. I'm getting 400 cc implants: Lukas Prantl and Martin Grundl, "Males Prefer a Larger Bust Size in Women Than Females Themselves: An Experimental Study on Female Bodily Attractiveness with Varying Weight, Bust Size, Waist Width, Hip Width, and Leg Length Independently," *Aesthetic Plastic Surgery*, vol. 35, no. 5 (2011), pp. 693-702.

97. Do Vietnamese bikers measure up?: Thomas Bell, "Vietnam to Ban Small-Chested Drivers," www.telegraph.co.uk, Oct. 29, 2008.

99. Debrahlee Lorenzana: Elizabeth Dwoskin. "Is This Woman Too Hot to Be a Banker?" *The Village Voice*, June 1, 2010.

100. Covering Your Assets: Sarah Anne Hughes, "Holly Madison Insures Breasts," *Washington Post*, Sept. 30, 2011.

101. Will I get better tips?: Michael Lynn, "Determinants and Consequences of Female Attractiveness and Sexiness: Realistic Tests with Restaurant Waitresses," *Archives of Sexual Behavior*, vol. 38, no. 5 (2009), pp. 737-745.

101. Carol Ann Doda: To read more, go to www.imdb.com/name/nm0230051/

CHAPTER 5:
Tits & Ask

114. How much does breast augmentation cost?: www.CostHelper.com, search for breast augmentation.

115. Don't think that medical tourism: Nancy Melville, "Weakened U.S. Dollar Brings Cosmetic Patients State-side," *Cosmetic Surgery Times*, Oct. 1, 2008.

117. Wanted: The Owner of These Breasts: "World Briefing/Germany: Police Hunt Breast-Enlargement Cheats," *The New York Times*, Oct. 5, 2006.

118. Can I deduct breast implants?: "Stripper Finds Support in Bust Ruling," *Los Angeles Times*, April 13, 1994.

118. Are implants marital assets?: "N.D. Supreme Court Mulls Value of Breast Implants," *Bismarck Tribune*, Dec. 3, 2009.

119. Carrie Prejean: Alan Duke, "Miss California USA Sued Over Breast Implant Money," www.cnn.com/entertainment, Oct. 20, 2009.

119. Navy: Nick Squires, "Australian Navy Pays for Breast Enlargements," *The Telegraph*, Sept. 17, 2007.

CHAPTER 6:
Surgery: Ready, Set, Go

123. Do I need a mammogram?: American Cancer Society Guidelines for the Early Detection of Cancer, www.cancer.org.

126. Cocaine With Your Surgery: Howard Markel, *An Anatomy of Addiction: Sigmund Freud, William Halsted, and the Miracle Drug Cocaine* (New York: Pantheon, 2011).

127. What's Your Favorite Number?: Alex Bellos, *Here's Looking at Euclid: From Counting Ants to Games of Chance - An Awe-Inspiring Journey Through the World of Numbers* (New York: Free Press, 2001). To take part in Alex Bellos' survey, go to www.favouritenumber.net.

NOTES _____

130. Her Breasts Were Seen by Thousands: Wang Qianyuanxue, "Chinese Dancer Blogs About Breast Implant Operation," *People's Daily Online*, Sept. 6, 2010.

134: Let Me Introduce You To: *The Tonight Show With Jay Leno*. NBC. June 19, 1997.

CHAPTER 7:
Recovery: Is That Normal?

141. A Housekeeping Service: Wang Yufeng, "Man With a Mission, License, Launches Into Ripe Breast Massage Market," *Global Times*, May 19, 2011.

146. Put Them to Work: Lauren Pyrah, "Bearing All to Panda to Charity," *The Northern Echo*, Nov. 28, 2007.

155. Natural Weapons: Busty Heart, *America's Got Talent: Season 3 Finale*. NBC. Oct. 1, 2008.

157. Unsnap, Separate: For a list of IG Nobel Prize winners, go to www.improbable.com/ig/winners. To buy The Emergency Bra, go to www.ebbra.com.

157. Saved By Her Sports Bra: Associated Press, "Sports Bra Saves U.S. Hiker Trapped in Alps," www.msnbc.msn.com, June 23, 2008.

CHAPTER 8:
The Three Rs: Raise, Reduce, Replace

161. Each year in the United States: ISAPS International Survey on Aesthetic/Cosmetic Procedures Performed in 2010, www.isaps.org, released Dec. 2011.

162. A study in the Aesthetic Surgery Journal: Brian Rinker, "The Effect of Breastfeeding on Breast Aesthetics," *Aesthetic Plastic Surgery*, vol. 28, no. 5 (Sept. 2008), pp. 534-537.

167. Cosmetic Breast Surgery Around the World: Colin Stewart, "16 Housewives, 12 Pairs of Breast Implants," *The Orange County Register*, Dec. 16, 2008.

168. The IDEAL Breast Lift: Ted Eisenberg, "Simultaneous Augmentation Mastopexy: A Technique for Maximum En Bloc Skin Resection Using the Inverted-T Pattern Regardless of Implant Size, Asymmetry, or Ptosis," *Aesthetic Plastic Surgery*, vol. 36, no. 2 (April 2012), pp. 349-354.

170. Never Too Old: Abby Ellin, "The Golden Years, Polished With Surgery," *The New York Times*, Aug. 8, 2011.

174. Greek physician Paulus Aegineta: Gordon Letterman and Maxine Schurter, "History of Reduction Mammaplasty," in *Symposium on Aesthetic Surgery of the Breast* (St. Louis: C.V. Mosby, 1978) pp. 243–249.

178. What happens when a silicone gel implant breaks?: Center for Devices and Radiological Health, U.S. Food and Drug Administration, "FDA Update on the Safety of Silicone Gel-Filled Breast Implants," June 2011, www.fda.gov.

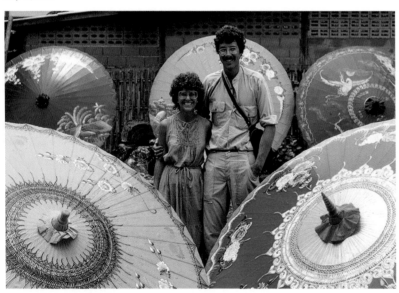

Long before he became a cosmetic breast surgeon, Dr. Ted had an appreciation for beautiful round objects. Above: Joyce and Dr. Ted admire handpainted silk umbrellas at a village shop in Northern Thailand in 1982.

CREDITS

Cover photo by Nuno Silva
©iStockphoto.com

Original Illustrations by Anoki Casey
Opposite Table of Contents, 10, 12, 15, 17, 19, 26, 27, 28, 37, 39, 41, 44, 53, 60, 77, 78, 79, 83, 85, 90, 95, 97, 98, 100, 102, 107, 111, 114, 127, 130, 132, 141, 144, 147, 149, 150, 153, 157, 159, 165, 168, 169, 173, 176, 178

Stock Photo/Illustration Credits
Inside Cover: ©iStockphoto.com/moonmeister
Opp. Title Pg:
  ©iStockphoto.com/thebroker (ice cream)
  ©iStockphoto.com/CAP53 (pinup girl)
Copyright Pg: ©iStockphoto.com/Lorado
Pg x: ©iStockphoto.com/karrapa
Pg xvi: ©iStockphoto.com/D4Fish
Pg 1: ©iStockphoto.com/TonyBaggett
Pg 2: ©iStockphoto.com/amoklv
Pg 4: ©iStockphoto.com/pinkpig
Pg 6: ©iStockphoto.com/Ka66
Pg 7: ©iStockphoto.com/karrapa (bras)
Pg 7: ©iStockphoto.com/temmuzcan (belly dancer)
Pg 8: From the collection of Sara A. Dreisbach
Pg 9: ©iStockphoto.com/LUNAMARINA
Pg 13: ©iStockphoto.com/MrPants
Pg 14: ©iStockphoto.com/nicoolay
Pg 16: ©iStockphoto.com/4kodiak
Pg 17: ©iStockphoto.com/kirza (crying baby)
Pg 18: ©iStockphoto.com/creacart
Pg 20: ©iStockphoto.com/ivan-96 (corset engraving)
Pg 20: ©iStockphoto.com/weareadventures (model)
Pg 21: ©iStockphoto.com/GreenPimp
Pg 24: ©shutterstock.com/zebra0209
  (Fountain of Diana)
Pg 25: ©SaraHodgson2002
Pg 22: ©iStockphoto.com/AleksandarPetrovic
Pg 27: ©iStockphoto.com/Nobilior (breasts in TV)
Pg 29: ©iStockphoto.com/aggressor
Pg 30: ©iStockphoto.com/allyclark
Pg 32: ©iStockphoto.com/Kontrec
Pg 33: ©iStockphoto.com/lovelens
Pg 36: ©iStockphoto.com/LockieCurrie
Pg 38: ©iStockphoto.com/Dphotographer
Pg 40: ©iStockphoto.com/logoff
Pg 42: ©iStockphoto.com/dddb
Pg 43: ©iStockphoto.com/cdwheatley
Pg 45: ©iStockphoto.com/thepraetorian

Pg 46: ©iStockphoto.com/cdwheatley
Pg 48: ©iStockphoto.com/filadendron
Pg 50: ©iStockphoto.com/IP Galanternik D.U.
Pg 51: ©iStockphoto.com/fitie
Pg 52: ©iStockphoto.com/duxpavlic
Pg 54: ©iStockphoto.com/Knaupe
Pg 55: Top Row L-R ©iStockphoto.com:
  Elfstrom, Lingdang, Lubilub, Miljko
Pg 55: Middle Row L-R ©iStockphoto.com:
  ValentynVolkov, Kazakov, akeeris, gdagys
Pg 55: Bottom Row L-R ©iStockphoto.com:
  xyno, 221A, RuthBlack, HamidEbrahimi
Pg 57 ©iStockphoto.com/twentyfourworks
Pg 58: ©iStockphoto.com/Dphotographer
Pg 59: ©iStockphoto.com/moonmeister
Pg 61: ©iStockphoto.com/MachineHeadz
Pg 62: ©iStockphoto.com/duncan1890
Pg 63: ©iStockphoto.com/Booka1
Pg 64: ©iStockphoto.com/karrapa
Pg 65: ©iStockphoto.com/xua
Pg 66: ©iStockphoto.com/JCStudiosLLC
Pg 68: ©iStockphoto.com/nailiaschwarz
Pg 69: ©iStockphoto.com/simonox
Pg 71: ©iStockphoto.com/b-d-s
Pg 73: ©iStockphoto.com/CandyBoxImages
Pg 75: ©iStockphoto.com/sjlocke (breast exam)
Pg 75: ©iStockphoto.com/A_N (couple)
Pg 76: ©iStockphoto.com/stockphoto4u
Pg 78: ©iStockphoto.com/AlexvandeHoef
Pg 80: ©iStockphoto.com/DanielBendjy
Pg 82: ©iStockphoto.com/stevendd (needle)
Pg 82: ©iStockphoto.com/Juanmonino (model)
Pg 84: ©iStockphoto.com/yew
Pg 88: ©iStockphoto.com/CollinsChin
Pg 89: ©iStockphoto.com/JuanDarien
Pg 91: ©iStockphoto.com/katikvi (4 illustrations)
Pg 92: ©iStockphoto.com/okeyphotos
Pg 93: ©iStockphoto.com/upheaval
Pg 94: ©iStockphoto.com/ru_
Pg 96: ©iStockphoto.com/Kate_Sept2004
Pg 97: ©iStockphoto.com/vinayaprashanth
Pg 99: ©iStockphoto.com/stevegraham
Pg 100: ©iStockphoto.com/ultra_generic (money fist)
Pg 101: ©iStockphoto.com/Vasko
Pg 103: ©iStockphoto.com/Lattapictures
Pg 104: ©iStockphoto.com/upheaval
Pg 105: ©iStockphoto.com/Lambada
Pg 106: ©iStockphoto.com/smt3

Pg 107: ©iStockphoto.com/cdwheatley
Pg 108: ©iStockphoto.com/LdF
Pg 109: ©iStockphoto.com/FreeTransform
Pg 110: ©iStockphoto.com/heather_mcgrath
Pg 111: ©iStockphoto.com/AlexeyBakhtiozin (fairy)
Pg 112: ©iStockphoto.com/katielittle25
Pg 113: ©iStockphoto.com/NLshop
Pg 115: ©iStockphoto.com/DNY59
Pg 116: ©iStockphoto.com/kickers
Pg 117: ©iStockphoto.com/CurvaBezier
Pg 118: ©iStockphoto.com/SaulHerrera
Pg 120: ©iStockphoto.com/MilosJokic
Pg 121: ©iStockphoto.com/ecliff6
Pg 122: ©iStockphoto.com/GrabillCreative
Pg 123: ©iStockphoto.com/MissMaudie
Pg 124: ©iStockphoto.com/Mervana (pill)
Pg 124: ©iStockphoto.com/dhanford (sick girl)
Pg 125: ©iStockphoto.com/ThomasVogel
Pg 126: ©iStockphoto.com/juhy13
Pg 127: ©iStockphoto.com/MindStorm-inc (bird)
Pg 128: ©iStockphoto.com/Brainsil
Pg 129: ©iStockphoto.com/id-work
Pg 130: ©iStockphoto.com/sceka (lady)
Pg 130: ©iStockphoto.com/nico_blue (theater seating)
Pg 131: ©iStockphoto.com/pchristinaq
Pg 133: ©iStockphoto.com/Vik_Y
Pg 134: ©iStockphoto.com/pick-uppath
Pg 136: ©iStockphoto.com/picturemaja
Pg 137: ©iStockphoto.com/lovelens
Pg 139: ©iStockphoto.com/dutchkris
Pg 140: ©iStockphoto.com/artjazz
Pg 141: ©iStockphoto.com/dee-jay (truck)
Pg 141: ©iStockphoto.com/Pimonova (mother & baby)
Pg 142: ©iStockphoto.com/MichaelSvoboda
Pg 143: ©iStockphoto.com/MichaelSvoboda
Pg 145: ©iStockphoto.com/juhy13
Pg 148: ©iStockphoto.com/pecopeco
Pg 151: ©iStockphoto.com/bluberries
Pg 154: ©iStockphoto.com/janedoedynamite
Pg 155: ©iStockphoto.com/fotokostic
Pg 156: ©iStockphoto.com/travelif
Pg 157: ©iStockphoto.com/SaulHerrera
Pg 158: ©iStockphoto.com/SaulHerrera
Pg 159: ©iStockphoto.com/friztin
Pg 160: ©iStockphoto.com/Viorika
Pg 161: ©iStockphoto.com/Ben185
Pg 162: ©iStockphoto.com/mocker_bat
Pg 163: ©iStockphoto.com/FurmanAnna

Pg 164: ©iStockphoto.com/BriArt
Pg 166: ©iStockphoto.com/vgorbash
Pg 167: ©iStockphoto.com/cimmerian (globe)
Pg 167: ©iStockphoto.com/CHR1 (Brazil)
Pg 167: ©iStockphoto.com/CHR1 (USA)
Pg 168: ©iStockphoto.com/-ALINA- (girl in box)
Pg 170: ©iStockphoto.com/Kativ (falling money)
Pg 170: ©iStockphoto.com/meshaphoto (ladies)
Pg 171: ©iStockphoto.com/stetanolunardi
Pg 172: ©iStockphoto.com/dumayne
Pg 173: ©iStockphoto.com/sdart (crane)
Pg 174: ©iStockphoto.com/evan66
Pg 175: ©iStockphoto.com/VeeDOK
Pg 176: ©iStockphoto.com/alashi
Pg 179: ©iStockphoto.com/hidesy
Pg 180: ©iStockphoto.com/multiart
Pg 181: Top Row (L-R) ©iStockphoto.com:
  bibi57, NilouferWadia, Will09, MichaelMerck
Pg 181: Middle Row (L-R) ©iStockphoto.com:
  siloto, arindambanerjee, amandalewis, lowball-jack
Pg 181: Buttom Row (L-R) ©iStockphoto.com:
  janedoedynamite, mixformdesign, hobu4ohok,
  AndraSimionescu
Pg 182: ©iStockphoto.com/BeauSnyder
Pg 183: ©iStockphoto.com/dedMazay
Pg 187: ©iStockphoto.com/Fitzer
Back cover: ©iStockphoto.com/asiseeit

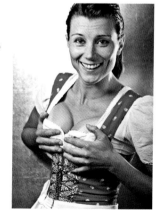

INDEX: Questions by Chapter

CHAPTER 4:
Size Matters

CHAPTER 5:
Tits & Ask

INDEX: Questions by Chapter _____

CHAPTER 8:
The Three Rs: Raise, Reduce, Replace

ABOUT THE AUTHORS

TED S. EISENBERG, D.O., FACOS, FAACS, is a Philadelphia-trained plastic and reconstructive surgeon and creator of the Ideal Breast Lift™. For the past 13 years at Nazareth Hospital he has focused his practice entirely on cosmetic breast surgery. He holds the Guinness World Record for the most breast augmentations done in a lifetime. He is on the faculty of a Philadelphia medical school and teaches his cosmetic breast surgery approach to doctors around the world. An inductee in the International Knife Throwers Hall of Fame, Dr. Eisenberg is ranked as an expert knife thrower and is nicknamed "The Boobinator." www.lookingnatural.com

JOYCE KIRSCHNER EISENBERG, a writer and editor, is a longtime contributor to Fodor's travel guides and the author of *Let's Visit Grenada*. Her writing appears regularly in *The Philadelphia Inquirer* and in newspapers and websites nationwide. Her 15-year stint as an editor at a Philadelphia Jewish newspaper gave her the chutzpah to co-author the *Dictionary of Jewish Words*; her stint as the doctor's wife for 30-plus years made her the maven to co-author this book. www.thewordmavens.com